GETTING MY HEAD AROUND ME

John Wise

To my darling Kel, for everything

CONTENTS

Title Page
Dedication

Chapter 1	1
Chapter 2	12
Chapter 3	21
Chapter 4	43
Chapter 5	50
Chapter 6	69
Chapter 7	86
Chapter 8	91
Chapter 9	106
Chapter 10	129
Chapter 11	136
Chapter 12	142
Chapter 13	148
Chapter 14	162
Chapter 15	167
Chapter 16	177
Chapter 17	181
Chapter 18	190
Chapter 19	197

Chapter 20	204
Chapter 21	212
Chapter 22	217
Chapter 23	221
Acknowledgement	241

CHAPTER 1

It was one of those eureka moments that occasionally occur in life. One where suddenly everything falls into place, the scales fall from the eyes, and you say to yourself *"Of course!"* The problem that I have had never even been considered by anyone, least of all by me, throughout the sixty years that I have been around on the planet, although I cannot think why, given my life's experiences and general personality traits. But then I have spent a career looking at others and trying to determine what has been causing the problems that they have come to me with. I have never really taken the time to look at my own life and reflect upon issues there. Which of us does? Such self-reflection in my profession would have been considered as self-indulgent navel-gazing and thus frowned upon until relatively recently. However, it turns out that I have had Asperger's all along. Or, rather, more properly, Autistic Spectrum Disorder (ASD. After a lifetime of wondering why I did not get what others got regarding social environments and friendships, of avoiding social situations where I felt overloaded and uncomfortable, of watching TV coverage of Glastonbury or passing a packed pub when the football is on and thinking "Why the fuck would you ever go there?", now I had an answer. After a divorce and estrangement from my children, one of whom definitely followed in my footsteps with regards to my personality traits, and a succession of difficult working environments and relationships, it all became clear. It's not just you, it's me too, of course it is, it always was. I never liked large groups, parties, or being the centre of attention. I was always self-reliant and did not seek comfort from others. I always took the view that a problem shared was a problem that two people now have. I was always a bit intense with what I wanted to do, and liked to develop my own routines, never really being comfortable if these were derailed or other people attempted to change them. In short, I was never really fun to be around, but now I know why. There are so many things in the past that suddenly just make sense, and so many echoes of those past events that still resonate today. As with many such conditions there are different levels of expression and mine is at the mild end of the range. My experience is therefore going to be different to that of others, but there may be others like me out there who have never considered that this might apply to them too as they are not severely affected. However, there may be recognizable traits that have led them to similar or recognizable situations and patterns of behaviour. So, let's look back together and try to understand in better detail just why I am where I am, and why I am who I am. Perhaps some of this will reflect your personality or that of somebody that you know.

In reading this book, please try to disengage judgement, and instead engage empathy. Just because I may have responded to situations differently to the way that you do, it makes neither of us right or wrong, just different. Let me give an example unrelated to neurodiversity. I am not a strong swimmer, having learned relatively late in childhood. I can do a reasonable breaststroke but cannot do a front crawl because I have never mastered the breathing technique required. Now some people reading this will say "Oh you too, I can't do that either!", whilst others will say "But the breathing is so *easy,* what's the problem?" And there you have it, different abilities. What is easy for one is difficult for another, and this is merely a mechanical action. Now transfer that difference in ability to one of perception and tolerance of the surrounding environment and hopefully understand that not everyone sees and perceives and manages the world around them the way that you do, but also that neither of you is the greater or lesser for that. The fact that neurodiverse people are in the minority does not make them wrong, just different.

I was the middle child of three and was born and raised in leafy Southeast London. Of course, it was not "real" London, it was

North Kent, but it was part of London's largest borough, and had the red buses and black cabs, so surely it counted. Bus travel was cheap and efficient, and us children got used to travelling around unaccompanied in our teenage years.

My name had been my mother's choice. My father's choice was to become my middle name, Edward, and I was pleased that I did not get that. It was bad enough when people found out my middle initial and said, "E for Ernie is it, Ernie Wise?" as if this were either amusing or original. I soon got fed up with the feeble joke but still tried to manage a smile each time as these people clearly considered themselves to be the greatest wit imaginable and this was the response required and got rid of the joker on that occasion in the shortest time. In my later career it would be replaced by "Wise, what a good name for a doctor", which was only slightly better.

The name John had been chosen as it could not be shortened, but it could be lengthened, which is typically a child's perverse response to being thwarted in one direction. It was therefore lengthened by my classmates to Johnny, causing much hilarity amongst other adolescent boys who felt that the subject of "johnnies" was suitably naughty and forbidden to be sniggered over at every opportunity, even if they had never seen a prophylactic device and were only vaguely aware of what they were for. Eventually it was my surname that won out and Whiz or Wizzy were the most common names I went by. To this day, whenever I have an inner dialogue, especially over some embarrassing or ill-judged event I refer to myself as Wizzy, whether to chastise or to encourage. It is also what my wife most commonly calls me, to my face at least.

Our family was financially secure but not well off, and, though we never went without the necessities, there were not too many extras. However, this realisation was retrospective, and we felt no deprivation at the time, it was just how things were and comparisons were never drawn with the apparent lot of others. I did experience, though could not remember, the great freeze of 1963, when the roads froze for weeks on end, and the milk was delivered by sledge, laboriously pulled by a muffled and behatted milkman up the slope to the estate from the gritted main road several hundred yards down the hill. At the time, we lived in a relatively modern bungalow heated by a fire in the lounge, and our own activity, supplemented by woollen layers, hot water bottles and eiderdowns. It is interesting to reflect that the family nostalgia includes such things as the freezing winter in detail, but no mention was ever made of where we were or what we were doing during other momentous occurrences that same year, such as the Great Train Robbery or the assassination of President Kennedy. It was the cold that made the greatest impact upon us, and our horizons were small.

We had no central heating back then, as was testified by the ice on the inside of the windows on winter mornings, the condensation not remaining liquid for long enough to run down and accumulate on the windowsill. There were two of us boys. The other one, the youngest of the three children, was christened Steven but was for ever known as just Steve. We used to chip off the frozen condensation and let it melt on our tongues. In fact, we were twins, non-identical and separated in birth by a mere ten minutes, but that still made me the older one. We were also quite different in appearance and character, such that people later would not have guessed that we were even related, let alone that we were twins. Between ourselves and our older sister, Louise, there was a gap of almost four years, meaning that she always considered herself superior and the three of us never spent any significant time together as a group. There was a single bar electric fire high up on the bathroom wall which was operated by a long cord which dangled from the side of the cylindrical heater, and which ended in a plastic acorn, but the room was still so cold that undressing to get into the bath, for there was no shower, was just as much of an ordeal as getting out again into the cold bathroom, there to steam furiously whilst trying to get dry on an already-damp towel and then get dressed again. The bath itself was cast iron under its coloured enamel, and was barely heated by the water it held, and so this did nothing to prolong the occupant's stay within. The lounge had French windows which opened out onto the garden and there was a dining area with table and chairs and a hatch through to the kitchen. At the other end of the lounge from the dining table was an open fire which burnt coal from the concrete bunker in the back garden. The bunker had heavy sliding hatches on the sides from which the coal was accessed by a small shovel and transferred to a tall scuttle that stood like a sentinel at the side of the hearth. There was a large hatch at the top into which the grimy coalmen would empty several sacks after carrying them in from the road on their shoulders one at a time. Steve and I used to love watching the coal truck pull up in the road outside the house, and then see the men alight and come around to the back of the vehicle. They would sling an empty sack on the apparatus there and then start the mechanism that sent a stream of shiny black coal into the sack with a satisfying whooshing sound and a small cloud of coal dust. It was more entertaining that watching the dustmen, for instance, who would clatter down the side of the house to empty the household dustbin into one of their own, and then carry that around on their shoulders to the truck out on the road and tip the bin up manually to empty the contents into the back. This was long before large, wheeled bins became available and had to be left out at the kerbside.

Our mother fought a desperate battle to keep on top of the laundry and there always seemed to be a line of washing blowing gaily across the width of the back garden. However, this was not possible when the weather was wet or cold and there were no tumble driers available then to use, so she used a folding wooden rack, or clothes horse, which stood in front of the fire. The washing machine was a twin-tub model, filled with hot water via a hose from the kitchen sink tap, with soap suds added to one tub that had a paddle fitted. This rotated one way and then the other to agitate the washing in the frothy water. There was clean water in the other tub for rinsing the washing afterwards. From there, the washing was lifted out using large wooden tongs, a piece at a time, and was fed through a hand-operated mangle to squeeze the surplus water from it, before being deposited on a metal tray on the far side. It was then moved to the spin dryer which stood upright, like a stubby space-age rocket with a lid, and a curious upright cylinder within, punctured like a colander. When switched on there was a loud click as the lid locked and then the whirring sound it made would gradually build in speed and volume until it seemed deafening, and the machine gyrated slowly across the kitchen floor as if it had a life of its own, depositing water from a spout at the bottom into a receptacle tied beneath it as it went. The receptacle had to be tied rather than just stood as the machine's perambulations across the kitchen meant that it would leave the receptacle far behind it and a trail of water would mark its progress across the tiles.

The bungalow was of red brick, was semi-detached, and was of a chalet style, such that all the rooms were on the ground floor except for the main bedroom which was situated in the roof and had a dormer window overlooking the garden at the back. The whole development had been built on the site of a former pig farm and so the land was rich and fertile and conducive to the home cultivation of fruit and vegetables, with which our parents supplemented the family table. For years afterwards we were aware that our parents would hold up fresh produce bought at supermarkets and state that it was not a patch on what they used to grow in Mater Road. Shopping was a daily event when we were young, with Mum taking her wicker basket and string bag and getting only what was needed for that night's meal, supplemented by additions from the store cupboard as needed. When we were old enough, we attended the local infant's school, which necessitated a good two mile walk each day from the age of five, as we had no car, or indeed any family member capable of driving at that point. There was also no bus route nearby at that time, though there was a bus stop near the arcade of shops by the school, and buses that stopped there could take us to the nearest town.

The shops themselves were different back then too. There were few supermarkets, if any, and those that existed were just large self-service grocers rather than the barn-like superstores so common these days. I remember the nearest example, a good bus ride away, which had a delicatessen counter on the way in where there was always a large ham in pride of place on a white porcelain stand, resplendent in its coat of yellow crumb, awaiting the administration of the carving knife by the attendant in response to the next order. There were separate shops for everything that one wanted, and the only two such examples that remain nowadays were the butcher and hardware store. The former has changed during my lifetime, though. I remember the tiled floor being strewn with sawdust, and rails with assorted items hung up on metal hooks. There would be whole chickens there, plucked bare except for around the head, with the hook supporting them pushed through the beak. In Winter months, items of game, such as pheasant or rabbit, would also be similarly hung, their numbers reducing steadily over the weeks towards Christmas. The staff would be wearing striped aprons bespattered with blood and various other detritus of their trade. There were also rows of large wicked-looking knives, as well as hacksaws and cleavers hung on the wall to be reached for to prepare a customer's chosen joint. Slowly most of this activity became hidden in the background and the shops themselves became gleaming areas of tiled sterility with packaged or pre-prepared meat. With regards to the hardware shops, I used to find them to be like an Aladdin's cave when I accompanied my father in search of nails, tools or other such apparently masculine items. They seemed to be labyrinthine places packed from floor to ceiling with goods and with tools hung and secreted in every conceivable space, and with the whole establishment being pervaded by a mixture of smells. The most overwhelming at the time was that of paraffin, which was used for domestic heaters and seemed to be dispensed with careless abandon and extraordinarily little in the way of modern health and safety precautions, but that was a smell that has long since been confined to history.

Fruit and vegetables were available at the greengrocer, whose establishment would burst forth from the shopfront every morning and colonise the pavement in front, with shelves of fruit stacked above floor containers full of the more robust vegetables. I remember how the shop assistant would dig into the pile of potatoes in one such container with the shiny curved metal bucket from the hanging scales to get a load which was then placed onto the waiting scale and subsequently added to or subtracted from by hand to get to the desired weight of produce for the customer, a process that usually seemed to end with the question from the grocer: "It's just over Luv – alright?"

The vegetables would then be deposited into the string bag that had been brought along for the purpose, smaller items going into brown paper bags first that were torn from a sheaf strung up on the shelving by a loop of string through their corners and subsequently closed with a deft twist of the wrist once they had been filled. Then there were the fishmongers, the last example of my more recent acquaintance having closed some years ago, with sloping white marble slabs containing a mixed shoal of various fish and other seafood in amongst the sea of ice which festooned the surface. A favourite Saturday experience when I was younger was for the family to go to Bromley by train, having first caught a bus to the train station. Once there we would wander along the high street and explore the various shops or stare into their windows at the goods displayed there. I remember how the streets changed with time and supposed progress, and the large Churchill Theatre being built in the High Street. I used to like the gardens behind the theatre, which predated it and were terraced with meandering paths through the mature shrubbery, a duck pond, and an amphitheatre. The gardens were a place of play and imagination for me and Steve as we charged around after one another, or hid in the shrubs, playing our games and trying not to get lost or too dirty. When I once returned to that place as an adult many years later, I saw that it would have been almost impossible to have got lost, given the small size of the area and sparsity of the planting, but the gardens had seemed an impossibly large wilderness to our young minds at the time.

These Saturday afternoon trips always included two compulsory stops. The first was a favourite butcher whose sausages were incomparable, apparently. They had two branches in the town initially, one at each end of the High Street. This may have had something to do with Bromley having two railway stations too, also with one at each end of town, up the hill or down the hill, Bromley North, and Bromley South. The underground network reaches to the former station now, but they were thought of as well out of London back then. The butchers were presumably placed for opportunistic purchases of something for tea on the way home, and survived on both sites for some years, until only the Bromley North shop remained. Eventually this, too, was swept away by the tide of change in the shopping sector, and those sausages are still mourned by my mother to the present day.

The last stop was at the fishmonger at the bottom of the high street, near the southern most of the two railway stations in Bromley, the one from which the train home would be caught. Here would be purchased some soft roe, a pair of herrings, or a kipper for my father's tea, and usually some golden haddock for us children. This was haddock that was dyed yellow and had a subtle smoky flavour imparted by some process that did not include the application of smoke, as true smoked fish was considered too strong and salty for our taste, no doubt correctly. Dad was always on the lookout for kippers that tasted like those of his own childhood in the New Cross area of South London, and those available at this fishmonger were, he thought, the closest thing to them. He liked his kippers grilled and then served with plenty of malt vinegar and white pepper, and with buttered brown bread on the side to mop up the juices and to help ease down the throat those fine bones that had been overlooked in his dissection of the fish. I still remember the smell of those cooked fish on chilly winter afternoons as the darkness drew in, with the wrestling being shown on the television, followed by the interminable football results. The wrestling would be the old-style combat of implausibly overweight contestants in swimming trunks and boots, rather than the gym-honed physiques and costumed personae of modern times, but the choreography and good-versus-bad characterisations were much the same.

In between these emporia in Bromley high street was the coffee importers, halfway along. There could be no doubt about what it sold as there was a working coffee-bean roaster in the window and an all-encompassing aroma of freshly ground coffee for some distance either side of the open doorway. It was a double-fronted shop and, whilst one window held the roaster, the other contained a working toy model of an ape of some sort that never seemed to tire of swinging over and around its wire support. Once over the threshold, there was a counter on the ground floor selling bags of ground coffee and boxes of pastries, whilst a flight of stairs up the right-hand wall took customers up to a delightful mezzanine haven of small tables with white tablecloths at which they could order any variety of coffee and patisserie. At a time when the coffee served in most establishments was made from a teaspoonful of granules or powder from an almost-empty catering sized tin and then topped up with hot water from a wall-slung urn, this experience was something special. At least, I took my parents' word for it, with me being of an age where a milkshake was much more the thing at the time.

I remembered devastating the vegetable patch in the garden with Steve when we took our little tricycles across it in a vain attempt to imitate the scrambling motorcycles that we had seen on World of Sport, and for which we were duly punished. We liked to watch the bikes, which sounded like angry wasps as they buzzed around the course and sent up sprays of mud whilst they climbed and twisted around a track that resembled the battlefields of the Somme, the riders ending the race caked with mud over their fronts with visibility limited to a small clear space on their hastily wiped goggles. Similarly, I remember propelling our scooter around the garden before flying off the single step in the middle where the garden level dropped, just to imagine I was really jumping on a motorcycle.

In all, I had happy memories of the family's time in that bungalow. It may have been the rose-tinting of nostalgia, or the fact that life was so much less complicated then, with satisfaction in simplicity being much more abundant and there being no thought or expectation of anything better. I spent my infancy and early school days there and watched as things in the local environment changed around me. A large council estate was built down the road and, although this had brought new schools and a better bus service with it, I missed the more rural environment that there had been, and especially missed watching and talking to the scraggy ponies that used to occupy the field before it was given over to dense housing and the blocks of flats.

School itself was a challenge. Steve just seemed to make friends at will whilst I struggled and never really found myself comfortable in the company of others. I declined to put my hand up in class if at all possible, and just liked to keep my head down. I played with one or two class-mates in the break times but never really met up with anybody out of school, preferring just to be at home. This was a pattern that persisted throughout my school life. I also remember some rather cursory judgements being made. For example, one day our class was lined up in the assembly hall and we were given a recorder to blow into in turn. I had never seen one before and just blew into it as requested by the teacher but was immediately told that I obviously had no musical potential and was dismissed, along with several others who could not immediately dash out a tune or meet whatever criteria were being used to identify potential musical talent. It did not feel like a particularly inclusive process.

CHAPTER 2

As us children grew, it became apparent that going everywhere on the bus was simply no longer practical. Our mother had taken driving lessons and passed her test, and when her own parents decided to drop from two cars to one when Grandpa retired, they passed his car onto our family to use. It was an old-style Vauxhall Victor, with maroon and grey two-tone paintwork, small tail fins over the rear light clusters, and chrome everywhere. There was a striking radiator grill that made the car look as if it had a permanent rictus grin. When the family got this, our first car, I can remember my father digging up the area next to the bungalow to lay crazing paving made from broken paving stones bought cheaply from the council and delivered by a large tipping lorry that made a lot of noise as it delivered its load at the kerbside with a whoosh and must surely have broken the stones up a little more than they were already. I remember the pavements back then being made of rows of large flat slabs which occasionally broke or were lifted by weather or tree roots and were subsequently replaced by a team of men from the council. They would lift the broken stone and replace it on its bed of sand with a brand new one, tapping that gently into level placement with a large wooden mallet. I now knew what became of those broken ones once they had been replaced. The fence panel in front of the now-paved area was cut and hinged to form a primitive gate, and eventually a garage was built there. This was made with concrete uprights that had grooves down facing sides, into which were slotted concrete panels which each overlapped the one below it like shiplap and kept the weather out. The car was then driven in forwards, and the correct placement to allow the door to be shut behind it was achieved by tying a tennis ball to a string and suspending it from one of the ceiling beams such that it just touched the windscreen when the car was far enough in. The handbrake would then be applied by pulling up a metal ratchet with a T-shaped handle at the top that ran parallel to the steering column. When the garage was built, some of the paving had to come up and the stones were broken down smaller and used to make a low wall with a double skin and soil filling the gap between for planting aubretia and similar tumbling clusters of colours.

Another strong memory that I retained from this time was of my trips to the barber, though why that should have left such a strong impression it would be hard to say. It was very much a traditional barber's shop, with red leather covering to the adjustable chrome chair, and a board placed across the arms of the chair for me and Steve to be lifted onto in turn. The barber was a short man with white hair and a blue short-sleeved jacket or tunic that he always wore over a shirt with rolled up sleeves, and a tie. What I mostly remembered was the severity of the haircut that we had to endure at the hands of this man, and under the watchful supervision of our mother. Images of Norman soldiers will give you some idea of just how short the hair was over the neck and occipital region of the head, and the top was a number two buzz cut. I also remember the closeness of his cut-throat razor that was sharpened by being stropped on a leather strip hung beneath the counter before being used to trim any stray neck hairs, followed by liberal application of talcum powder from a small maroon and black rubber bottle that puffed the talc out when squeezed. In later years Mum always claimed that this style was for neatness, but we felt convinced that she had a fear of us coming home with nits, and so the style was designed to offer no chance of a grip to any passing head louse. I never remembered either of us having an infestation of lice though. However, that hairstyle is very much in fashion and now called a skin fade, so Mum was clearly just ahead of her time, although the current styles allow for considerably more hair to be left on the crown than Mum tolerated. I am sure that I remember Dad musing that perhaps the barber had some Native American heritage in him somewhere.

There were also some memorable neighbours at Mater Road.

There was a couple called the Pitmans to the right of the bungalow as you looked at it from the road. Steve and I would go there after school some nights once Mum had returned to work. At that time, she worked part-time as a school secretary, mostly because of the school holidays when she could be off for childcare, but also because the working day was shorter than in an office. However, she could not always get back home to be there when we boys got home from school, and so the Pitman's stepped in to help. We might occasionally have tea there but were usually just entertained until our mother got home. I remember that Mr Pitman often wore a soft collar around his neck, presumably because of arthritis, but he explained it at the time by saying that he had spent too long going around looking at the ground for pound notes.

To the left of the bungalow were the Humphreys. I remember them as an elderly couple but their grown-up son lived with them and was in his mid-twenties so they cannot have retired for long at the time. I can remember the Lambretta scooter that their son rode to work, and that Mr Humphrey also grew vegetables and fruit in his back garden but to such an extent that there was little room for lawn or flower beds. Indeed, such a considerable part of the length of the garden was given over to them that he seemed to be almost self-sufficient and was forever to be seen trudging back to the house with armfuls of produce. The features of their garden that I most remember were the wasp traps. We now recognise that wasps' chosen prey usually consists of insects that are seen by gardeners as pests, but Mr Humphrey had several jam jars placed around his plot, with jam residue left on the insides, holes punched into the top from the outside so that the distorted metal formed an inward-facing flange, and a sump of water reaching half-way up the inside. The idea was that the wasps would be attracted by the jam, crawl through the hole into the cavity of the jar, and then be unable to get out and thus eventually fall into the water to drown. There always seemed to be a reasonable level of accumulated corpses at the base of each jar, and Steve and I gave them a wide berth when we ventured into the back garden to retrieve a ball from our play, an all-too-frequent occurrence as the gardens were separated by chain link fencing just three feet high. As the football was made of leather and very heavy, especially when wet, Mr. Humphrey was extra-ordinarily tolerant of the damage the balls' frequent incursions did to his horticultural enterprise.

My earliest memories are of this house and the time we spent there just seems to merge into one long recollection when I try to look back now. It feels like a time of contentment and safety punctuated by occasional trips out, of family teas at various relatives' houses, and a progression through infant school. This latter was forward-thinking as it had its own swimming pool, but I did not see this as an advantage. The pool was an above-ground affair and was completely open to the elements during the time that Steve and I were there. I hated swimming and just remember shivering uncontrollably and wondering why we had to stand around outside in the teeth of a brisk breeze whilst soaking wet. It might have been considered as good training for seaside trips in the UK, as the general opinion back then was that there was nothing that a howling gale and horizontal rain could do to spoil a good trip to the coast, but I was sure that this was not the intended curriculum, and I did not learn to swim during my time there.

When Steve and I were eight, our family moved to a larger house several miles away. This was a semi-detached four-bedroomed house with a mock Tudor frontage, having dark-stained fake beams attached to the stuccoed exterior, and which was just down the road from a station on the main line into Charing Cross station in London. It was prime commuter territory, although my father still had to get to work by using two different buses rather than using the railway. However, the main reason for the move was to have more space generally and so that Louise, Steve, and I all had a bedroom each. The house was from the 1930s' building boom and was of a construction that had thick but single skin walls, with metal casement windows, parquet flooring, and a lounge and dining room separated by sliding doors, but these were solid rather than glazed. The lounge had a television in the corner, an electric fire in the chimney hearth, and a brown carpet with a peculiarly long pile. This quickly looked crushed by the passage of feet, and after vacuuming one had to use a plastic rake to bring the pile back up to make it look neat. After such administrations I always thought it looked like a ploughed field. The lounge also had French windows which opened out onto a crumbling patio, beyond which was a long narrow garden with a huge silver birch tree halfway down the right-hand side. The dining room overlooked the front garden. In this room there was a record player to the left of the chimney breast and a display cabinet to the right, which had white frontage and smoky glass in the doors above the drop-down drinks' cabinet door. Our mother's indispensable tea trolley stood proudly in the opposite corner next to a low sideboard in teak. Sunday tea was taken in the lounge and was made up of sandwiches, crisps and a freshly made cake, all brought through to the lounge on that tea trolley, which still occasionally gets pressed into service.

There was a coal bunker at the edge of the patio, and a small shed with a corrugated asbestos roof just beyond it. The bottom half of the garden had a path which was almost circular enclosing a round bed with three conference pear trees in soldier formation to the left-hand side, and a small compost heap beyond.

From the back gate there was a passage that ran down the side of the integral garage, and which led past the back door, just beyond which was an outside-facing cubbyhole or coal shed. No doubt this had pre-dated the coal bunker but was no longer used, and eventually Mum and Dad arranged for a builder to block up the door and knock down the interior walls to enlarge the kitchen and give room for a breakfast table there. They had central heating installed, after much cursing and sweating by an unfortunate plumber who had to do battle with the thick walls using an electric drill which seemed to be nowhere near up to the job. He preferred crawling under the suspended flooring to run pipes rather than having to drill through too many walls. This system used a gas boiler and so the old solid-fuel version went, along with any point in retaining the coal bunker. Eventually this was dismantled and removed to enlarge the patio space outside the kitchen window and improve access to the shed.

The house move meant that we were much closer to all shops and services, except for our schools, which remained tantalisingly distant, but still walkable and so we walked there and back every day. Unlike the bungalow, there was a good parade of shops just at the top of the road, set around a turning circle for buses. The centre of the circle was an island which housed an estate-agents and a large pub. The move had come when we were one year into our Primary Schooling and the new school that we had to attend seemed to be an improvement on our old one. There was an Infant and a Junior School sitting next to each other, but across the road from the Infants School was the old primary school site, which was still occasionally used for its classroom space and playing fields and was known as The Annex. These buildings were all of wooden construction and decked out with very old-fashioned door and wall fitments of a sort that I recognised many years later when working in hospitals and had to venture down to some of the older parts of these buildings. The Annex has since been demolished and the land used for housing. The new school was bright and spacious and had the unbelievable luxury of an indoor heated swimming pool. Behind the school was a thin strip of woodland with a stream running through it which was occasionally accessed during lessons to show aspects of the natural world. That same stream could be accessed further along outside the school property and was a favourite site for some of my own nature exploration. The one other thing I remember was a particular teacher at the school. He was never my form teacher but that did not seem to matter. At the end of break time all pupils had to line up in their forms before being allowed back into the building one form at a time. It was then that teacher came into his own as he would prowl up and down the lines looking for anybody who was doing anything he could consider as naughty and then step in and mete out punishment. He wore a never-changing outfit of brown suede desert boots, ill-fitting grey trousers, and old shabby tweed jacket, unkempt facial hair, and an expression of undiluted vitriol. If he decided that somebody had done something wrong then he would administer a hard slap around the back of the head or to a bare leg, for we all wore shorts at that age, and would make the miscreant stand out front and wait to go back into class late. There were usually several such miserable souls at each break time. However, there was no further punishment for being singled out. I was once caught out possibly talking or fidgeting, or just breathing in an overly antagonistic way, and duly received a clout to my occiput from a hand which then propelled me to the front. However, when I arrived slightly late back to my class I received just a look of slight pity from my form teacher and no further mention of the incident was made. It seemed as if this teacher was just permanently in a rage against some misfortune in the hand that fate had dealt him, possibly in the sartorial department, and he just took it out on the pupils at the school at every opportunity just because he could. The other teachers just seemed to accept that this is how he was. I am not sure that he would get away with that these days.

Steve and I were put into different classes in this school at the behest of our parents, who wanted us to be judged independently by our teachers and not just thought of as "the twins" where we might be judged as a collective. Steve did his usual Pied Piper act to attract a flock of friends, whereas I struggled and perhaps made one or two. I occasionally used to kick a ball around the park or play some cricket with them but was never really tight with anyone, preferring my own company and activities most of the time. I suppose that this is my earliest clear memory of how I was and how I liked to spend my time, and how I seemed so different to my brother in this. I did not see it as a problem at the time, although I think my parents, having separated us at school to avoid making comparisons, then did exactly that at home regarding our social activities and all that separating us at school really did was highlight the gulf in social skills between us.

My parents were keen to try to enforce some kind of engagement upon me, and I suppose I wanted to please them, but it always ended up with us both being disappointed. The boy scouts were a case in point as they were keen for me to join. I was somewhat reluctant but had the usual line from them that I would enjoy it once I was there. I didn't, of course, but then I had to "give it time", and then a uniform was purchased so I felt some kind of obligation to continue to go, but I hated it. I managed to persuade them to let me stop after a year, but they were clearly disappointed in me. It was as if they had read a manual of things that boys like and wanted me to do them, without ever actually asking if they were things that this particular boy liked. Steve never went to scouts so presumably he was deemed to be doing sufficient "boy stuff" already. I was content with solitary pastimes and my own company, but I presume that this did not appear in the manual and so it was ignored.

There was one, occasion, though, when quite the opposite happened. I always liked to listen to Radio 1 as a teenager, and I used to like to listen to the Radio 1 Roadshow that was on over the summer months back then. A production unit travelled around the British coast, broadcasting a show every weekday morning with a different presenter each week picked from the ranks of the usual presenters on the station. It was a live show broadcast from some open site at whichever town they were in that day, with a crowd of local resident and holidaymakers just turning up to be a part of the action. I really wanted to go to one of these but there was never an opportunity except just once. We were on a family holiday in Devon at the same time as the roadshow was in that part of the country. Better still, they were to be broadcasting from Plymouth on the same day that our parents had decided we would visit. It was surely fate! But when I asked if I could go, the answer was a definite "No!" Apparently we were to be touring a gin distillery that morning, which was not particularly engaging for a young teenager, and

I missed my one opportunity to see the show live. Worse still, our afternoon itinerary was to walk across the Hoe, the large area of open ground near the sea and the site from which the show had been broadcast. By this time the crowds had dispersed, and the Roadshow trailer sat isolated and forlorn, all closed up and waiting for the crew to get back from the pub and tow it to the next venue. Mum even pointed it out and asked if that had anything to do with that show I had kept going on about. I could have hit her, I honestly could. She and Dad had repeatedly pushed me towards things I did not want to do because they thought I should be doing them, but when it came to something I really wanted to do, and I did not ask for much, it had been denied to me because it was inconvenient. What was a couple of hours out of one morning of my life compared to a year of bloody Scouts, but I hadn't been allowed to attend. Looking back, I do not know how I would have been in the crowd, as I had never been to anything of that nature before, but my natural tendency would probably just have been to hang out at the fringes. I would still have liked the opportunity to have experienced that event though.

CHAPTER 3

The change of home meant that bus and train travel became much more accessible, with a choice of bus routes and the train station less than a five-minute walk away. This was mostly beneficial to us children, however, or on trips to London, as the family did now have that Vauxhall that we had acquired at our previous address. This was just one of a succession of variably reliable second-hand models that came and went through my childhood, and it meant that no journey of any length was entirely without an element of jeopardy as to whether the car would get to our destination and back without throwing a mechanical hissy fit of some sort.

These vehicles were all driven by my mother as my father had once tried driving and decided he was temperamentally unsuited to it. Rather than follow any kind of instruction, or the Highway Code, he wanted to do it his way, and that required that everyone else on the road be made aware of that fact and make suitable allowance. If he had lambasted fellow users as a driver in the way that he did as a passenger, then there would surely have been a series of accidents caused by his inattention. Of course, there were no compulsory seatbelts at this time, and no rear seat belts at all, so the consequences of any accident could have been severe. Dad, having lost confidence in all cars after our various experiences, spent most of any journey looking at various dials in the dashboard relating to revs and oil pressure, tapping them violently to ensure they were not stuck, and then diving under the dashboard to investigate some extraneous noise, real or imagined, which he considered to be a harbinger of impending breakdown. How our mother got anywhere unscathed with all this distraction, and variously inaccurate map-reading, is anyone's guess. The refrain of "That road we just passed, that was the one we needed to take!" was all too common, and usually followed Mum's warning of an impending junction with a directional decision to be made, only to find that Dad had removed his finger from the relevant part of the Automobile Association Book of the Road so that he could impart some uncomplimentary comment about a fellow road user.

Our father worked in purchasing and supply for an industrial manufacturer, and one of my abiding childhood memories was of the gifts received by our household at Christmas time from company representatives in thanks for that year's business and trying to curry favour for the coming year. Dad would come home with bottles of alcohol, each one disguised in its own conical hat of straw as protection as this was in the days before plastic bubble wrap was around. My father was not a big drinker, and certainly not of the whisky that was the gift that he most received, and so he had come to an arrangement with the owner of an independent off license up the road from where we lived. Almost every business was an independent concern back then and so the owner had free license to make his own decisions. He would take in Dad's surplus, knowing that he could easily sell them on, and exchange them for bottles of things that our assorted relatives preferred on visits to the family home over Christmas. Dad preferred Pernod and Campari, and bottles of port, advocaat and vermouth were duly brought home in place of the unwanted, but clearly very marketable, whisky. Sometimes there would be large hampers delivered into which we could delve amongst the straw and shredded paper to find exotica such as boxes of macadamia or pecan nuts, tins of pate and coffee, and jars of pickles or preserves, as well as exotic tea, chocolates, and assorted condiments. These were things that did not normally feature on the weekly shopping list and often held pride of place in the pantry all year, untouched and out of place, being saved for a special social occasion that never seemed to arrive.

On one memorable year, Steve and I were treated to a racing bike each by some enterprising rep who clearly wanted to think creatively. We each had a bike at that time, with normal flat curved-back handlebars, and rode on these across all terrains, from road to recreation ground, through woods and down tracks. However, one day near to Christmas we got back from school to find that waiting for us in the kitchen, resplendent in orange paint and with white-taped drop handlebars, were two brand-new racing-style bikes which represented unbelievable luxury and not something that either of us had ever dared aspire to.

Before we moved up to senior schools there was the Eleven Plus exam to be taken as a selection process which was used to sort the supposed academic wheat from the more practical chafe. I duly passed and found that I had been assigned a place at the local grammar school. Although referred to as local, it was a good four miles away as the crow flew, and further still by road. Fortunately, I got a lift to and from school with my mother who was still in the same job as a school secretary at a different establishment, although I could walk to my new school if needed and I often did once older. After all, I had walked two miles to the Junior School on all but the wettest days when younger and we were all used to walking to get about. There was not so much of the school run phenomenon back then and being dropped off at school or collected afterwards was quite a rarity. Steve, incidentally, had also passed his Eleven Plus, but the headmaster at the junior school persuaded our parents that he would be better off at a more practical school, given that was where his perceived strengths lay, and he should not, therefore, also attend the grammar school. Given that Steve fell among a crowd at his subsequent school that tended to drag him down and away from study, such that he barely scraped a couple of CSEs, I wonder whether he might not have done better in a different environment, and I am concerned at just what an impact that headmaster's opinion had on Steve's whole life.

The grammar school was quite a modern building, like the junior school I had attended. It was a long-established institution with its origins in Tooley Street, near to London

Bridge, and it had relocated within the recent past. The school had originally been founded during the reign of Elizabeth I, and this historical connection was celebrated by an annual memorial service every Autumn in Southwark Cathedral, in whose shadow Tooley Street lay. This major undertaking involved decamping the whole school to London, walking us from the school premises to the local train station, supervising the rail journey, then walking again to our destination, keeping us all quiet through the service, and then getting us back to school again by reversing the journey. No mean feat for the staff who somehow managed it every year with only minor casualties sustained.

The site of the relocated school was now suburban and surrounded by playing fields and trees, and the new school building had a bold red brick frontage which included an angular chapel of striking design with feature windows of bold stained glass, and a tall spike on the top. The whole chapel stood on stilts at the front of the school and was joined to it by a short glass walkway. The school made much of this feature and of having a resident chaplain, but our family were not church-goers and I never really understood what confirmation was, let alone why some of my contemporaries would have confirmation classes on top of school. The school was low rise with two floors, and there was an architectural nod to the old school in that most of the classrooms were set around a large quadrangle, edged with walkways bounded by brick pillars. During break times the enthusiastic and active younger pupils often used to play running games across this space and between the pillars and many a cup of coffee was knocked from the hands of unsuspecting teachers as they made their way from the staff room to their next lesson after break, with curses and detentions being as liberally spattered about as the coffee. During their morning breaks the more senior boys were to be found in their common room upstairs just starting to nurture their own caffeine habit.

Although I had managed very well in junior school, I found the going a bit tough in the second and third years at grammar school. I struggled with some of the concepts and found that I did not deal well with not being on top of the work set by the teachers. My end of term report cards made increasingly dismal reading over these two years, until suddenly something seemed to click in the fourth year and things seemed to hang together and make a lot more sense. This was especially true of the science subjects which all seemed to flow into each other in a coherent and understandable way. Quite why this happened I do not know or question, but I just seemed to "get it" whereas previously the subject matter was just grey and indecipherable. I was never great at languages, although I somehow managed to carry my rudimentary knowledge of French vocabulary with me for decades afterwards. I was OK at mathematics but was happier with the baser concepts of algebra and geometry rather than calculus, which I never really got to grips with. Of the sciences, physics always seemed more elusive than the chemistry and biology that I was happier with. I did not know if the physics issue was its reliance on mathematics, or was down to the teacher, who made much of the boys needing to explain the basis and theorems used behind their answers, but, when correcting them, would make no such references himself, and so learning was a little limited. It was a poorly kept secret that this teacher liked a quick sojourn to a pub down the road at lunchtime when possible and this may have had something to do with his shortcomings.

My other great love was art. I particularly liked pencil or water colour and, though not great by any means, I had always found that I could usually make a good enough representation on the paper of what I saw or imagined, and I was thus encouraged enough to enjoy it. I have dabbled with this skill throughout my life, and I was even able to get an extra A level examination in art just by doing a little coursework and a couple of pieces when the exam time came.

One thing that I hated at school was any activity that involved acting or performance. At grammar school, an ability to perform on the stage was considered every bit as desirable as a penchant for rugger. No doubt the captains of industry that they expected us all to be would need to be adept at public speaking or controlling board rooms full of committee members. Each class had to perform in turn at morning assembly, and each teacher had to ensure that every boy got a turn at being involved. Whilst this approach might have helped a recalcitrant or shy youngster to "give it a go" at Junior school level, on older children it had the opposite effect. Instead of helping me to discover a hitherto unknown love of the stage, it merely deepened my hatred of it.

I remember one Christmas disco at Junior School which was held in the classroom at the end of term when I was sufficiently carefree to attempt to replicate what I had seen dancers do on the television. I also remembered two or three other boys at the side of the room pointing at me and laughing, and also how I felt about being singled out for this treatment. I never did anything like that again and have remained self-conscious about dancing ever since, as well as avoiding anything where I might be seen and singled out for negative comment. This was a feature that I noticed over the years, whereby I might try things, but I would avoid repeating anything at which I had experienced disapprobation, either real or imagined. Another example of this at Junior school was when Steve and I were playing soccer for our house team, and I scored a goal. I was not going to mention this at home as I never liked to draw attention to myself, but Steve did. Dad therefore had quite a bit to say about how he expected that I did a couple of laps of honour and passed the cap around. If he had just said "Well done" or given me a pat on the back or thumbs up, that would have been great. However, his sardonic attempt at humour put me right off ever being in that position again. At the next soccer session, I volunteered to go in goal. I was not particularly good, but then neither was anybody else, including the incumbent at the time. This was probably because we were eight years old and defending a full-sized goal and so the chances of us being in the part of the goal where a kick was aimed were roughly the equivalent of the probability of an electron orbiting a nucleus being in a given point in space at a given point in time. The goalkeeper at the time grabbed with both hands the chance to get out from between the posts, probably the first thing he had grabbed with both hands for some time. I remained in goal until the end of my time at Junior School, witnessing lots of goals, but not scoring any, and not saving many either. Any successes that I subsequently had at Grammar School I then kept to myself. On later reflection I realised that Dad probably meant no harm by his comments and would probably have been upset if he had known how I had taken them. Similarly, most people would probably have shrugged off or immediately forgotten about his comments, but I am not made that way. My social armour is not strong, and the wrong word or gesture can pierce it easily and find some vulnerable place beneath. Similarly, I did not spend my life seeking my father's approval and mostly just keep my head down.

Whilst at grammar school too, I discovered that although I liked sport, and was passably good, I could not deal with how it was played. There were rules to follow for each sport, and follow them I did, but I noticed that nobody else did and, indeed, the assiduous following of the rules was positively discouraged if that meant not winning. The heady ideals of playing the game and it not mattering whether one won or lost simply did not apply. The attitude espoused was very much that winning was everything, meaning honour and prestige for the school, and seemingly anything was allowed in the pursuit of that end. Cheating, or "gamesmanship" as it is euphemistically referred to, was the order of the day, in much the same way that "business" is the term often used to describe one person taking financial advantage over somebody else who is not able to fight back, rather than being a commercial exchange from which both parties benefit. However, this attitude struck at the very heart of my sense of right and wrong, and I could simply not deal with that. Although I was of a reasonable standard and even played rugby for the school a few times, I could not deal with the negative and persecutory attitude of others towards me for playing the game properly and losing, rather than winning at all costs. Neither could I accept the culture that was developing around the sport as we got older, related to bawdiness and, later, the absolute requirement for inebriation after the event. This was bad enough during sixth form at school but became worse when I got to university where I found that standards of behaviour dropped even lower as the players got older, with one university rugby team even having the tag line of "Are you man enough to act like a child?" That and the tales of various unsavoury initiations into university sports teams of all sorts made me determined to avoid involvement and remain a spectator. I was not prudish enough to think it should not occur, each to his own, but I just did not want to be included and so I voted with my feet.

I was picked to play rugby for the school a couple of times because I could run and side-step a bit and scored a few tries in the games played in lessons and inter-house matches. However, there was no real coaching beyond the idea that you run forwards and pass backwards. For the first two matches I was in the backs so was part of a running line and knew where I had to be. However, for the third game I was picked to play full-back for some reason. I had no idea how to play that position because I had never been told, and the strategy and field positioning for defence and attack were mysteries to me. I also seriously doubted that I could kick to touch from anywhere significantly in-field from the touchline, which would be a necessary skill in that position. I therefore felt that I could not really cope with this on top of the stress of actually playing, which was already building each time I knew I had been picked. I also knew that there was no point in approaching the sports staff about this because they would not have given the tiniest of shits about it, so I backed out by feigning illness and, to my relief, was never picked again.

This was another attitude that defined me throughout my life. It opened me up to ridicule and to being considered unfriendly, a stick in the mud, or even just an outsider. In America I would have been thought of as a nerd, as I was certainly not a jock. However, this obsession of mine over playing fairly and by the rules was clearly part of an overall personality that manifested itself in many other ways too through my life, especially a fixation upon order and rationale and a dislike of chaos and irregularity, and which I did not identify for what it was until recently. This manifested itself in other ways too as I got older and made me vulnerable to others taking advantage of that. I was usually put down as being chronically shy or socially awkward and the true issue was never identified or even suspected. Indeed, although Asperger identified the condition that bore his name in the 1940s, it was not popularly used in mental health circles until the 1980s, so it was never going to be identified in my youth. It is only more recently that the nomenclature has changed to ASD.

There was also an incident in the sports department that opened my eyes to the casual laziness of authority that I recognised in all aspects of authority and bureaucracy later in life, but first came to my attention there. It was in the year of school when O levels (now called GCSEs) were due to be taken. Up until then, sports lessons were regulated into swimming lessons indoors, with outdoor sports being rugby in the Winter, or cricket and tennis in the Summer. Inclement weather in either season led to gymnasium work instead. The school decided that a little freedom was warranted at the age of sixteen and so a range of sports was available to fill up the games' lessons on the curriculum. Apart from the gym, weights room, swimming pool, tennis courts and playing fields, the school also has squash courts and even courts for curious game called Eton Fives. This uses a concrete court, similar in size to a squash court but with a buttress protruding from one side wall. Padded gloves are worn and used to propel a very hard ball instead of using racquets. Actually, only the palm is padded, and one soon learned not to strike the ball with the fingers as the pain caused was significant. Whilst this sounds great, this arrangement had obviously descended into chaos in the past with boys going to anything they fancied, leaving some sports ignored and others being oversubscribed. No doubt lessons had been learned and so the games staff dedicated the whole of the first double lesson to getting all the boys in the year together in the assembly hall to choose what they wanted to do in order that they then stick to that choice so that facilities and equipment would be appropriate for the numbers attending each activity. Each pupil had to name a first and second choice activity from those available, and, after the best part of an hour of list making and bartering, all pupils left the meeting knowing what they were going to do during their games' lessons for the next term or two. At least, that was the plan.

I had elected to do basketball, being quite tall and not without some ability to pass and shoot from most parts of the attacking half of the court. However, on the first lesson, it was clear that there were more boys present than had been expected. It was obvious too, exactly why that was, at least to the pupils. A group of friends had clearly decided that they fancied basketball instead of whatever it was that they had previously chosen, even though they had not been named in the basketball group when the decisions had been finalised. The solution was, of course, quite simple. The staff had the lists of participants for each group, and they could easily have consulted them and identified who should have been there, and then directed the interlopers back to where they were expected to be. However, they did not do that. The reason seems to have been that this group of four or five were "likely lads" who knew how much they could be cheeky and answer back without getting punished for it and could then have a jokey relationship with the staff. Clearly the staff running basketball thought they would have a better time for these lads being there, and so they went about choosing who should be allowed to stay in such a manner as to ensure that this group met the criteria. I was one of those who was to be disappointed and was told to leave. Of course, the only spaces left were those abandoned by the group in the first place, in an activity that I had no interest in or aptitude for, so I left the department and went to the library instead, where I spent every other games lesson for those two terms. After all, I had been crossed off the basketball list but not added to any other list, so nobody was expecting me to be anywhere. I found it exceedingly difficult to understand why the staff had not just done the most obvious thing to sort out the problem, followed their own rules if you like, but instead had shown favouritism and a casual disregard for anyone else. My need for order and rules did not compute with this on-the-hoof variation and the whole affair just struck me as unfair. Of course, this was a significant life lesson to learn, and I gained much more experience of such uneven supervision in managing all manner of situations in later life. I learned that having authority did not imply that one knew how to use it, or even care much if they abused it. Indeed, some people clearly aimed to get authority just so they could abuse it to make themselves more popular with certain elements. It was to be a recurrent theme that people in authority failed to follow the proper protocols and procedures in place, whether through laziness, incompetence or a vested interest in a particular outcome.

Although not participating, I still enjoyed team sports as a spectator, particularly rugby, which I much prefer to football. However, I never formed an affiliation with any individual rugby club, just preferring to enjoy watching the skill involved, whilst tending to route for whomever was the underdog in that fixture. I had found that when people supported a particular team, then their view of the match was adversely affected. If the other team did well, then they tended to bemoan the lot of their own, rather than appreciate the good play of their opponents. Although my friends would vehemently deny this, I felt that my point of view was supported when the NFL games of American Football started to be televised in the UK in the late 1970s. My friends and I would appreciate the spectacle of the new game, and highlights such as the thirty-five yard "bomb" pass for a touchdown, the long running play, and the defensive "sacking" of the opponents' quarter-back when he was caught in possession of the ball and was duly buried beneath a minor landslide of muscle, padding and testosterone. It did not matter who was playing, it was just thrilling to watch. But soon, however, favourite teams began to appear amongst my schoolfriends, merchandise for them became available by mail-order, and the same partisan attitudes that spoilt other team games for me, started to develop.

I view sport in the same way as art, as something which can stimulate a response in the observer, so why not enjoy it that way? Would one ignore Van Gough because they happened to like Rembrandt? And what about Canaletto, Titian, Constable, Turner? Are these to be off limits too? Did one route for watercolour and eschew all things oil or pastel? It just did not made sense to me at the time, and, to this day, it still does not. I would still prefer to just enjoy it for what it was, rather than have any emotional attachment to a particular outcome, though I can see that I am in the minority in having that view. The herd mentality and the ancient tribal default of "us against them" would both endure long past any counterargument that I could raise.

I have always maintained a satisfactory level of fitness throughout my life, but I have done this in a solitary way, using running, walking, weights, and yoga, and I was never keen on gyms or classes. When the latter became available to stream on-line much later in life, then I would participate, but I still preferred to do this alone rather than even joining Suzy, my wife. I did dip my toe into team sports once more, much later in life. A local private hospital used to host an annual cricket match between a team of local consultants and one of local GPs, a limited overs match with a wonderful barbecue and free bar afterwards, intended for professionals to meet in an informal way. I thought I would give it a go one year, envisioning a pleasant good-natured game and some convivial company afterwards. How wrong I was. Both teams seemed to be made up primarily of men who had excelled at cricket all of their lives and many still played for local clubs. However, there were too few of them to muster a full team of each and so the lower batting orders had a few like me just looking for a game. Still, all seemed OK at first and my low place in the batting order meant that I did not face any of the lethal-looking bowling during our innings. During their innings, the consultant openers were seeing off all the bowling, and so I was therefore put at somewhere between short leg and mid-wicket to apply some pressure to the batting. Sure enough, a good length delivery caused a mis-strike which sped my way at ankle height. I got down quickly and got both hands to it, but the ball was spinning viciously and managed to climb back out of my cupped hands before I could close my grip, from there to fall harmlessly onto the turf. My captain offered commiseration, but I could see he didn't mean it. Perhaps he had forgotten that decades of consulting with patients makes us experts at non-verbal communication, so whilst his voice was saying that it could have happened to anyone, his eyes and demeanour were saying that I was a wretch of the lowest order and that, far from laying a consoling hand on my shoulder, what he most wanted to do was to frogmarch me behind the pavilion and lay into me with a horsewhip, or possibly hand the job over to his fast bowlers whose upper limb musculature was no doubt better suited to the job. I kept my head down in the outfield after that but was allowed one over of bowling at the end, from which the winning runs for the consultants were scored. Far from being the captain's offer of friendship, I think he just did not want any of his good bowlers to suffer that ignominy. Instead of enjoying a convivial barbecue and a couple of drinks afterwards, when stumps were drawn, I fled, never again to don the white flannel garb. I also never put myself forward for the other event that this hospital hosted, which was a clay pigeon shoot. Somehow the idea of pissing somebody off that much whilst they were in possession of a loaded shotgun did not appeal.

I was never one for extra-curricular activities. There were many societies and clubs that met during lunchtimes and after-school, but I never wanted to be a part of them. I did my work at school, and my homework afterwards, and that was it. I did not look for more and was never particularly sociable, preferring my own company much of the time. Although I did have a small circle of friends, I did not even really see even those outside of school. I would always prefer to try to adapt some sport so that I could play it on my own, rather than try to engage in a team event of any kind. One of the ways that I did this was to use a tennis ball and a cricket bat. I would use an underarm throw to propel the ball against the wall of the house or shed and then treat the rebound as bowling, which I would then defend or bat away. I developed scoring systems for getting the ball to certain parts of the garden or down the side of the house, which required a particularly accurate cover drive. I would happily spend some hours at this but knew I would face utter bewilderment from my father who would wonder aloud how I could waste so much time "just patting a ball about" and why didn't I "go and have a proper game". However, in later life it became apparent to me that Dad himself had never taken part in team games, so it was puzzling why he had not identified that I was of a similar disposition, or perhaps he did and was trying to herd me in a different direction from that which he himself had taken. If this was the case, then it never worked, but it might have helped me to appreciate at an earlier age just how similar my father and I were. Instead, I did not seem close to my father as whatever I did, I just seemed to invoke his displeasure. He did have a dry sense of humour and told good jokes, but he also had a temper under which the pilot light was always lit which meant it could flare up quickly and unpredictably, so it was often easier not to be in his company. He had no passions or hobbies to share with us or pass on, so there was no real reason for us to spend time together, and he always seemed to have something that needed attending to at the weekends. Sadly, although I can remember Steve and I playing football and cricket with Dad when we were very young, I have very few memories of father-son occasions after that. Of course, that might be mostly my fault. When I was going to scouts, I brought home a flyer one week which advertised a Father and Son Day, in which there would be teams of each competing against each other in a variety of tasks and activities. I just brought it home as I did everything, knowing that there was no way I wanted to do that, and presumed my father would not either as he had never shown even the slightest inclination to do so. However, he seemed to grasp this opportunity with both hands and was all for it, possibly believing that this was just the sort of thing that I should be doing as a boy at my age. I was horrified, but my hesitancy was quickly over-ruled by the parental veto and so it was arranged that we would attend, with me getting more and more anxious as the date approached, because I knew that I would be overwhelmed by that whole environment. In the end I feigned illness on the day and so we didn't go, but later that day Dad came menacingly close to me and growled "Don't you *ever* do that to me again!" Of course, I didn't. Instead, I ruthlessly vetted anything that was to be brought home and removed anything that might bring about a repeat of that situation.

I was always interested in natural history. I would devour books and magazine articles on the subject, and, not surprisingly given my enjoyment of solitary pursuits, I would venture forth on my own outings, and had a particular fascination with water. Nowadays, a boy out alone in woods and off beaten tracks would cause a sharp intake of breathy alarm from most parents, but these were contrasting times, possibly a little naïve as tragedies did still occur, but they were not thought of as day-to-day threats to oneself and most parent were glad to let their children out from under their feet at weekends and school holidays. I would cycle off, with a dipping net strapped along the crossbar of my bike, and a jam-jar with string tied around the top as a handle swinging from the handlebars, to go and wander along the course of various streams and see what I could find. I would often bring back trophies to keep in a tank and watch for a while, before returning them to where I had found them. These could be sticklebacks and newts, frogs and their spawn, caddis fly larvae crawling along the bottom of the tank in their manufactured coats, water boatmen rowing invertedly across under the surface tension, and various other assorted creatures. The spawn I would often keep in order to watch its transformation into tadpoles, and their own subsequent metamorphosis as limbs grew, tails shrank, and body proportions changed. I would then return the now amphibious offspring to their original intended home. I often thought that my later interest in science and, ultimately medicine, stemmed from these excursions to satisfy my curiosity about the natural world around me and, at one point, I was determined to become a marine biologist despite being a poor swimmer all my life. Although this phase passed, I never lost my fascination for the natural world, and I have continued to enjoy articles and documentaries on the subject.

I also enjoyed comedy. I was never particularly fond of slapstick, and I enjoyed the re-runs on the television of Laurel and Hardy films for the confusion and wordplay rather than the joke violence and pratfalls. A good example of this was in one episode where the two of them were driving around residential streets in a small truck from which they sold fish, and Stan gave Ollie an explanation as to why they should have their own boat and catch their own fish to sell and thus make more profit, rather than buying it from a fisherman to sell on. In the sketch, he gets the explanation right first time, at which Ollie is so taken aback that he asks Stan to repeat it. Of course, this feat was beyond Stan, and he tied the various elements of his explanation up in inextricable knots trying to do so. I was a bit young to appreciate the Goons and Round the Horn, especially as the latter relied too heavily on Polari and double entendre for my tender years to understand, but I subsequently discovered the brilliance of Monty Python and was one of those boys who would learn long parts of the script to disgorge at opportune moments. But it had to be right. All the words had to be correct, as well as their delivery. Python did that to people. Even following the death of Queen Elizabeth II when King Charles III was processing through the streets and protestors could be seen holding placards stating such things as "Not my king" and "I didn't vote for you", my immediate thoughts were of Monty Python and the Holy Grail. There is a scene when King Arthur is trying to explain to a peasant that you don't vote for kings, but that the lady of the lake had held aloft the sword Excalibur, thus showing by divine providence that he was chosen as king of England. In reply, the peasant states that

"Supreme executive power comes from a mandate from the masses, not some farcical aquatic ceremony" including some "moistened bint lobbing a scimitar."

I have since pondered but could not identify any modern equivalent to Python. There was The Fast Show with characters such as the car salesman stating that everything in life bore a relationship to lovemaking, or a ramshackle character appearing from an outside shed door and stating that their recent diet had consisted mainly of an unlikely ingredient such as taramasalata. But surely these engendered a repetition of individual catchphrases rather than lines of brilliant script, and these other programmes did not encourage the wholesale learning and repetition of soliloquies and sketches, the way that Python did, back in the day. The nearest thing had been Fawlty Towers, which obviously involved one of the Python team. Of course, there were no videos or on-demand access to anything then, so books of scripts and the repeated listening to long playing records were the only ways to hear the material over several times and thus hope to remember any of it. This was made harder by my parents considering the whole genre "silly", ironically mimicking one of the colonel characters in the series itself, and thus banning it from the evening watching at home. Nobody had a spare television set in their bedroom at that time where they could have watched what they liked, and so that particular avenue of pleasure was cut off from me, as Basil Fawlty might have said.

Most of all I like dry humour, puns, wordplay, and the clever use of language. Stephen Fry's unmatched style of using complex yet accessible language appeals, and, like Fry, I have never tired of re-reading the stories of P. G. Wodehouse, especially the Jeeves and Wooster stories. Try as I might, I can never remember the phrasing used afterwards, but it makes me smile or laugh out loud every time I read the stories through and the carefully selected phrases leap from the page at me, every word used having been chosen to add just that extra touch of colour to the phrase without cluttering it up and spoiling the effect. It is pure artistry. There are similar examples of the craft in Dickens. Although they are sown more sparsely in amongst the evocative social commentary, the fact that Scrooge thought that there was "more of gravy than of grave" to account for his seeing Marley's ghost was one such example. Examples were scarcer still within Shakespeare, but they were there, wonderful phrases, economically painting a picture for the imagination, but they took much more endeavour to flush out from the dense woodland of prose in which they lurked.

Back to humour, and I feel that the pinnacle of the craft came in a sketch with Peter Cook and Dudley Moore. I have always found their comedy a bit hit and miss, in all honesty, but it did bear repetition in the same way as Python material, and there were wonderful highlights such as the parody of the summing up of the Jeremy Thorpe trial by Sir Joseph Donaldson Cantley, as well as the sketch I have in mind now. It featured the two protagonists sitting in an art gallery, dressed in rain-macs and flat caps as was their want, with packed lunches before them. I remember hearing comments from other comics about Peter Cook's brilliant mind and razor wit, but also how he would just go on talking at times, not necessarily being particularly funny but looking for the sharp punchline in a situation, rather like a champion boxer, possessed of dexterity and fancy footwork, with a lightening jab and devastating right cross, but still sometimes forced to slug it out until he found an opening through which he could land the knock-out blow. At one point in this sketch, Dudley Moore found Peter Cook's comedy getting the better of him, and, in an attempt to prevent himself from bursting out laughing, he tried to bite into the food before him. Cook, spotting the bulging cheeks and heaving shoulders of his partner, without hesitation quipped "You're really enjoying that sandwich, aren't you?", thus tipping his hapless colleague fully into the pit of helpless mirth. The timing, the dry delivery, and the economy of words was simply perfect. What a knockout punch that line was.

Another clever use of wordplay was between the double act of Armstrong and Miller who had a series of sketches featuring two World War II pilots who spoke with clipped upper-class accents but in a modern patois. It seemed to me that this was actually an extension of a Monty Python sketch about a collection of similar pilots, who spoke in a form of banter common at the time, but who could not understand each other's comments, such as "hairy blighter dickie-birded" or "cabbage crates over the briny", if they ventured into the Officer's Mess of another airfield. But the juxtaposition of educated voices and street vocabulary was equally pleasing, having just exchanged one sort of banter for another. This paring also did some other parodies which I enjoyed. The first was a singing double act that was clearly based upon Flanders and Swann, but instead of singing about glorious mud or a ninety-seven-horsepower omnibus, these songs started out bawdy and became increasingly rude, until they were invariably cut off as if some censor had pulled the plug. The other was the character of a television historian played by Ben Miller, who would demonstrate some rare item, cradling it in gloved hands and describing its provenance in hushed tones, ending by saying that it was, of course, "absolutely priceless," at which point he would accidentally set some series of actions in motion that would destroy the artefact. This was the nearest thing to slapstick that I could relate to. I always think that the measure of good comedy is that it still makes you laugh even when you know what is coming.

The other form of comedy that I grew to like was observation comedy. What I remember from when I was younger, was that a comedian was somebody who stood up on stage with a microphone and told jokes, describing a situation, and then giving a punchline, usually in terms that would be considered misogynistic or discriminatory by today's standards. My father also used to relate his experiences of music hall or variety show comedians, such as Max Miller, with rapid fire delivery and risqué content. However, the idea of pointing out the amusing and ludicrous elements of everyday life was not so common. The first exponent of this that I noticed was Billy Connolly, who came along during my teenage years. The use of terms that described bodily functions, and the pointing out of certain behaviour appealed to my sense of humour, as did the recognition that his comments applied to observations of my own experience. This became more apparent during my medical training, when the observation of patients featured significantly as part of the diagnostic process, and I would notice idiosyncrasies and differences even more but could never have highlighted them in the same amusing way. However, the appropriate use of Anglo-Saxon terms for bodily functions was very much a part of my future career as technical or medical terms invariably went right over patients' heads, and I found that an interested stance was easier for patients to engage with than a judgemental one. I suppose the most popular recent exponent has been Michael McIntyre, with many people being able to identify with subjects such as differing gaits in different circumstances, and the fact that many households in the land, including ours, have a male member who purloins some area of storage in which to deposit what Suzy refers to as accumulated crap. However, I don't understand a routine that he does in which he says that, now being of an age where he has to get up at night to urinate, and not wanting to disturb his wife by putting the light on, he goes into the en-suite facility and does his best with his aim, invariably missing the pan and the consequences of that. Just sit down, Michael, for God's sake – you can't miss then! It's not rocket science.

The last comedian I shall mention was Victoria Wood, who combined the elements of the observation of life's minutiae with the clever use of language and colloquialisms and thus effortlessly covered both bases.

As I grew into my teenage years, it became apparent that the aspirations of my parents for the next generation to do well, sat squarely on my shoulders. I was no genius, but I coped comfortably with schoolwork once past that sticky patch in the middle senior years, being helped by a good memory, and that watershed moment after which I understood and enjoyed the science subjects. I also was able to retain much of what I was taught if I went about it in a particular way and strung it all together.

Though also intelligent, my siblings were distracted by the other diversions of teenage life, and they did not attain anything significant academically. Despite this, they were still subsequently able to make a path for themselves through life, my sister working in a bank and human resources before working for Formula One, and my brother getting a mechanical engineering apprenticeship after leaving school.

I therefore became determined that I should do my family proud and vowed not to do anything to cause my parents further anguish. What with my older sister having an eclectic variety of boyfriends, and my younger brother being out with a gang of mates and occasionally fighting in the streets, I thought that they had enough to cope with. Because I was usually at home whilst my siblings were out during school holidays I was put to work by my mother. I would have to peel vegetables, lay the table for meals, help clear away, and then wipe up the dishes and cutlery after Mum had washed up. My siblings managed to breeze in just before a meal, and then sidle away immediately afterwards without offering any input at all. I was convinced that my mother was using household chores to try to force me into social life that I did not want and was not looking for. Instead, all I did was rankle at the unfairness of it all. This attitude of putting the preferred outcomes of others before my own aspirations or immediate desires became a habit that I found impossible to break, and certainly made me open to manipulation as I got older. When I married Suzy and was asked by her "What would *you* like to do?" I found it impossible to answer. I was so used to either not being considered or trying to second guess what the asker of any such question actually wanted me to say, that I found it impossible to state clearly my own preferred option in any situation. It was several years before Suzy was able to coax an opinion from me on any matter, and she went out of her way to allow me the freedom do pursue that, even if it was just watching the rugby on the television with a pint of ale beside me.

I later found out that it was my father from whom my academic abilities probably mostly came, together with many traits of his personality, which seemed to germinate slowly and eventually burst forth into prominence later in life. Perhaps they had always been there, but I lacked the self-reflection of maturity and so did not notice them at the time. No doubt they were apparent, but which of us ever sees ourselves as others do? Certainly, I felt that my parents sometimes thought my behaviour odd but put it down to shyness. My father had also passed his eleven plus when younger and thus had also been bound for grammar school. However, he had been born one of seven children in a poor part of inner south London, with a father who had been a porter at Covent Garden fruit and flower market, now long since converted to a complex of retail outlets and bistros near the Royal Opera House. Money was therefore always tight, and his parents simply could not afford the uniform which was an absolute requirement for his attendance at the grammar school. Simply because of this shortfall he was forced to forfeit his place and subsequently left school at fourteen to enter the world of work, such was the hindrance to social mobility at the time. To a certain extent, that hindrance still exists, but hopefully it is not so stark. It seemed to me that Dad had wondered ever after just what his life might have been if things had been different, but I only gleaned this by its being hinted at in the odd phrase or reminiscence from time to time, and Dad certainly did not bemoan his fate. However, it clearly pleased him to see his son achieve a grammar school place of his own and be able to put it to effective use.

CHAPTER 4

It was uncanny just how much like my father I became as I matured in adult life, something that seemed more obvious to me than to others, strangely. There was even an errant patch of hair on my right temple that was like an area of my father's hair which I remembered seeing and that was placed identically and behaved similarly. When I became middle-aged the area developed an identity of its own in that it was greyer than surrounding hair and had a distinct concave wave that defied my hair-dresser's attempts to tame it to lie flat with the hair that surrounded it. Left too long and it would wave extravagantly but cut too short and it would bristle indignantly from the side of my head. Quite why that characteristic was genetically determined was a puzzle, but I had clearly inherited that particular gene and it both amused and comforted me at the same time, especially as it became more prominent after Dad's death and as I aged. Only recently Steve saw an old photo, in which Dad must have been around forty years old, and he had commented how much I currently look like our father did in that photo. Meanwhile I had watched myself gradually transform into a close semblance of my father for the past decade. I had slightly more hair, slightly fewer pounds, and a few more people skills, but otherwise the similarity was remarkable. Even my gait is like his, as he always strode along with a vaguely military air and sense of purpose about wherever he was going, even though he had been medically exempted from service during the war because of a heart murmur and so had never had military training.

I could have done with a little more of the fatherly input from Dad at times though. When I had my own son, I thought that a teenager was like an "apprentice dad" and needed to have some coaching in some of the things that dads did around the property and in life, albeit heavily weighted towards my own experience rather than that of dads more generally. I could have done with some tuition in shaving, for example. I had caught glimpses of my father with a face covered in shaving foam, vigorously rinsing off a yellow disposable razor in the sink full of water as he methodically removed the foam and bristles from his face with the razor. This was a process that always seemed to end with the application of several small pieces of toilet tissue over bleeding points. My own first attempts to shave were attempts to copy this process, augmented by some magazine articles that I had found. However, razor burn and nicks in the skin were still frequent attendants to my ablutions until I was older and had a cut-throat razor shave performed at a well-known Mayfair establishment where one descended the stairs to a haven of wood panelling and submitted to tilting chairs, hot towels and facial emollients before the bristles were removed by a keen blade, and where advice was liberally dispensed instead of toilet tissue. Shaving has been a much more enjoyable experience since then.

I learned the rudiments of decorating, gardening and simple carpentry by observation and copying, occasionally being allowed to use off-cuts of wood to try things with. We also learned Dad's Law of Do It Yourself, which was that in any project, no matter how large or small, there was always one *bloody* screw that refused to budge from where it was, or go into where it was needed, and that this would make the whole job last twice as long as was necessary. It was amazing just how often that law applied. As I became a teenager and thus stronger and more useful, I was pressed into service with heavy digging and the like, and I helped my mother to relay the entire patio and front drive with crazy paving, with me mixing the concrete and heaving the slabs about, and Mum using her eye for levels and pattern. It was a good job well done by the end of that.

I felt my parents' expectations keenly and I wanted to do well for them as well as for my own satisfaction. I was therefore a little perplexed when they seemed to be encouraging me away from this end throughout my teenage life. They would repeatedly ask why I did not go out at all with my friends from school, or whether I even had any. Why was I not interested in having a girlfriend like other boys or my brother? The fact was that I was simply not interested in that social element. I had always been happy in my own company and with my own ideas and interests and was never at a loose end or at a loss as to what to do. As for girls, I attended a single sex school and never did anything that might take my path across that of girls, so I simply never met any and was not looking to do so. The fact that the way I filled my time was different to most of my peers did not exercise me as much as it seemed to do to my parents. Looking back as an informed adult, I can identify the Asperger's characteristics with a predominance of social awkwardness, my level of self-reliance, my preference for order and routine, a tendency to take things at face value, and apparent rejection of others' input. All these elements remain with me to this day and assessments done have supported the theory. Of course, this condition would not have been recognised back in my childhood at a time when so many subtle, and not-so-subtle, nuances of personality and behaviour went unrecognised and thus also went unaided. However, the pressure to conform was there and I had detected in my parents' attitude the idea that there was something not right about me, they just could not identify it or confront it. It did occur to me that they thought that I might have been homosexual, which might have horrified them as they were from a much less enlightened era when it was against the law. Possibly they did not pursue their enquiries into how I chose to pass my time too vigorously lest they accidentally run some unpleasant quarry to ground and then not know what to do with it. It was one of the many things that were just not acknowledged in the family, let alone talked about.

When I was a GP later in life, I found that it was not that unusual for a child to be diagnosed with ASD only to have the child's mother come forward and point out that the child's father showed similar traits. The gender predisposition for the condition meant that it was less commonly the other way around. The father in question would often have had a tortuous and uncertain family, educational and employment history and be considered as stupid, rude, arrogant, disruptive, or, at least, "strange", unless they had managed to stumble upon or create a niche that suited them and their personality characteristics. For example, one such father had managed to cope with his difficulties by finding a job as a hotel night porter, where he was less likely to have to deal with many people or be exposed to too much sensory stimulation, which could overwhelm a person's abilities to cope if they had that condition. I have often wondered how many other adults there were out there, labelled as difficult or stupid because of their inability to engage with the "one size fits all" education system, and drowning in the morass of expectations of the general population unless they managed to secure a lucky foothold. I can remember a line from an elderly character in a Victoria Wood comedy about how dyslexia had not been heard of in her time at school but some children who did not do well with literacy were sat at the back of the class with some craft or other to amuse them. Similarly, there was no Asperger's mentioned in my day. Instead, children were labelled as "quiet," "shy," "a loner," "sensitive", "socially awkward," "a bit of an introvert," "not a good mixer," or most damning of all, "not a team player." How many promising intellectual futures were damaged by that phrase on a school report or work reference, and how much that was labelled a mental health problem or unsociable behaviour was just sensory misperception or personality that did not fit in with social norms? And who decided what those norms were? If somebody could not change how they saw or interacted with the world, why should they be labelled and judged by others? I have certainly seen my fair share of such problems in the course of my work, and I have always tried to explain the issues involved and look at what were reasonable expectations for the patient and those concerned about them. Actual help, should it be required, was unfortunately very sparse, but sometimes just the knowledge of why people were as they were, and that it was OK to be like that, was all that was needed.

When I was lecturing at university, I became aware that the incidence of dyslexia in the UK is around 10% of the population, rising to 20% of those at university. Fortunately, there was a lot of academic support and adjustments made to help those students with dyslexia to make the most of their educational opportunities. The incidence of ASD is around 1-2% of the general population, rising to 2.4% of the university population. However, the rate of drop-out from university of that demographic is around 40% of those students. This is surely an un-necessary loss to higher academic achievement caused, not by lack of intelligence or ability, but by a difficulty in fitting in with the prevailing social environment. There is so much more to the university experience than just attending lectures, and I cannot help but wonder whether students on the autistic spectrum would not do better if there was some kind of support available to help them with that environment, seeing as academic support so clearly benefits students with dyslexia.

I remember in my own father the traits that I subsequently recognised in myself and then, later, I saw that these also appeared in my own son. It was always the case that my mother was chatty and lively and could get on with anyone anywhere, whilst my father kept much more to himself and avoided unwelcome conversations with strangers if possible. He had no interest in their lives and could see no good reason why they should enquire about his. Interestingly, this exactly mirrors the reasons why I have no social media presence myself. I see no reason to give a running commentary of my life to others and have no interest in a running commentary on theirs, though I can see how the platforms might be useful for a rapid dissemination of information, for example. I feel that social media posts are a bit like those round-robin letters that everybody used to put into their Christmas cards back in the eighties and nineties. The problem is, they really only ever showed what they sender considered to be their best life.

The parents were devoted to each other and were either being promoted or receiving some other plaudit for their hard work, whilst the children were head pupil, or school team captain, or on a short list for a Nobel prize, or similar. Nobody's life is unrelentingly positive and golden and yet this is how the majority of these author's letters made their lives out to be, and how most of the lives that are documented in social media posts are made to look. Not for me thanks.

Dad could tolerate family and friends, but only in small doses, and he maintained a small, and not overly close, circle of friends. He had no hobbies or pastimes that brought him in touch with others and he did not seek out any form of social intercourse. This caused some tensions between my parents at times, especially once us children had left home. If they went anywhere, my mother would end up chatting to all and sundry, grateful for the opportunity to socialise, whilst my father would retreat to a corner behind a newspaper and not venture out, either physically or conversationally. Unfortunately, as so often, instead of recognising these traits in each other and accommodating them, they each tried to get the other to be like they were themselves, which was never going to be a productive strategy. Again, with hindsight, I realised that this may have been the cause of tensions in my own first marriage too, in that I shared my father's social intolerance of others, but I was not particularly good at articulating to my then wife, Rebekah, exactly why this was. She, on the other hand, was all for partying and having people over and clearly thought that I was just clipping her wings un-necessarily. On walking into a room full of people that I do not know, my natural tendency is to hug the wall and circle warily whilst looking down to avoid eye contact. On many occasions I would never get even that far. I would attend somewhere having said that I would, but not get beyond putting a hand on the door before feeling too daunted to proceed and thus retrace my steps and avoid the whole situation. At least I could be truthful and subsequently say that I had been there, although I might also use one of those old standbys, "It was shut", "There was nobody there" or "I must have got the wrong day" – possibly not so truthful. In extremis a drink was always helpful in a crush as one could be looking into it and thus avoid catching anybody's eye accidentally. One had to look somewhere and there would be people in every direction, so down was the best option. If I could sit at a table looking downwards then I would, and the eventual use of a mobile phone certainly helped with this. I then did not seem out of place if I was glued to one. Indeed, a mobile phone has become a lifeline for those of us with ASD who find themselves adrift in a sea of humanity.

I have managed to cope with this lifelong trait, and, although it has seemed to improve with age, the basic problems and behaviours have remained. It may just have been that I got used to coping with it and became more adept at avoiding situations where it would be an issue. I wish that I had understood it more when I was younger as I was constantly trying to be like everybody else but failing and not realising that I could not be like they were anyway. I always had this feeling that there was something I should be doing and was that I was missing out as a result but did not realise that this apparently tantalising prospect was never within my reach. As a middle-aged man I eventually learned to be comfortable in my own skin, and just point out that this was who I was, and that others must take it or leave it. It might be that I was different from many others, but not everybody was gregarious, the life and soul of the party, and it is certainly true that the pattern of life is made up of light and shade. Contrasting personalities make for a more interesting human experience overall, even if that did not necessarily include the dinner party or other social occasion that one was currently attending. However, I had focus, concentration, and determination, and that saw me do well enough to go to medical school.

CHAPTER 5

Quite why I chose to study medicine I never really knew. I was looking at biochemistry or marine biology initially, or possibly architecture. There was nobody medical in the family, except a cousin who had trained to be a nurse, and I had shown no particular predilection for medical matters before. However, I had done some voluntary work on a hospital ward on Sunday mornings, and I had found that I was comfortable both in that environment and with chatting to the patients and staff, which was quite a surprise to me as I was normally so reticent in social situations otherwise. It also applied later in my career when I was consulting with patients and so I decided it must be that I was in a particular role in which the rules of engagement were, in many ways, already set, so I could relax a bit and thus those elements of myself that were there could emerge rather than hide behind the terror of the situation and the need to initiate some interaction. There was no need to impress, and an agenda was already implicit. Over the subsequent years I had many compliments on my bedside manner, and the fact that I was prepared just to listen to what people had to tell me, without jumping in or interrupting, and I found this all the easier as I was genuinely interested in what patients had to tell me because it helped me determine what the problem was. I was sifting the information gathered and searching for clues in the detective work that is medical diagnosis, and the need for me to understand exactly what was being said helped me to take a good history as an important part of that process. Whilst some might consider me a pedant, I always like to be sure I understand exactly what the patient is trying to tell me, as it is all too easy to jump to conclusions and fill in the gaps incorrectly.

When the time came for university applications, I did notice that the dearth of extra-curricular activities on my application forms worked against me. Universities wanted captains of sports teams, wide and varied social interests, political engagement, or leadership opportunities, and they would use the lack of these and other such excuses for wielding the scythe when cutting down the plethora of applications to a number that could manageably be interviewed. I visited and applied to several medical schools, and all of them were far enough away from London that I would need to leave home to attend, as I somehow felt that a break from the family home environment was important. I could not have explained quite why that was the case even to myself, but I determined that this was a necessary step. I was offered only one interview but was fortunately offered a place on the back of that. More importantly still, having once left home, I never really went back to live there again. This was no conscious choice, just the way of circumstance as university life led straight into professional life in which I had to be resident in the hospitals where I worked, but in doing so I preceded my more worldly siblings in flying the nest by several years.

I continued to enjoy art, particularly drawing but I dabbled with water-colour on occasion. I had been told that I was good at drawing since childhood, and I just enjoyed being able to represent what I saw on paper. I was not excellent, and would never make an artist, and it gave me much enjoyment over the years, though it tended to be a pass-time that waxed and waned with time, with me having bouts of activity and productivity, and long fallow spells in between. However, again, I found it useful in my career when explaining things to patients. Long before I learned about different learning styles as a university lecturer, I had noted that the adage of "a picture paints a thousand words" was absolutely true when trying to simplify and explain complex medical or anatomical issues to some patients. I found that a pad and pencil were just as important as a stethoscope to have available in my GP consulting room most days.

Doubtless because of my general personality and social

awkwardness, my sexual awareness was more than a little under-developed. As mentioned, I had not had any experience with girls as a teenager, primarily because I had gone to an all-boys school and had no social life to speak of. However, in an attempt to earn some money of my own, I had done a Saturday job in an electric light shop, and it was not long before the male shop manager kept trying to feel me up. This was my first contact of a potentially sexual nature of any sort. I was seventeen at this point and uncertain what to do, but I knew that the attention was unwelcome and thus my parents' potential concern about my sexual proclivities was clearly unfounded. By this age I was large and strong enough to physically defend myself if required but I was uncertain if that was what was warranted here and so I looked for another way to deal with the unwelcome advances. I was the only shop assistant and the shop manager concerned was married with children, although a little camp in mannerism, and he clearly had broader tastes than his marital situation would suggest. I made my unwillingness to cooperate known, at which the manager sulked hugely and practically ignored me, then slowly tried to wheedle his way back to the status he felt that he had before I had said this. Of course, looking back I should have told my parents, confronted the man and threatened to report his behaviour which was clearly a sexual assault, or possibly just punched him on the nose the first time he tried it and walked out, but then it was all a mystery, and such things were hardly ever heard of and never spoken about. There was also the concern that it could be thought that I had somehow invited this behaviour. I had left a previous weekend job at the local branch of a large national supermarket because I was so shocked at the childishness of the management staff. They treated all weekend staff as imbeciles and took petty delight in deriding them and giving them pointless tasks to do. It did not sound as if they were any better with each other, and I once overheard one telling another about how he had tripped a colleague up in the toilet and then urinated on him. I presume he considered that to be funny. However, my leaving that job was a decision that sparked significant concern amongst my parents because of the money I was turning my back on, so I did not want to let them down again. And the five pounds a week that I was paid for working all day on a Saturday in the light shop was certainly useful, though a little stingy, especially as I had to pay my train fare there and back out of it. In the end, I managed an uneasy truce with the manager until my A levels were over, and I could escape to university, feeling that this was another life lesson duly learned.

Once there, I floundered at first in the strange environment, feeling totally overwhelmed with so much that was new. Despite me wanting to make the break, I was dreadfully homesick to start with, even though I was living in a hall of residence with plenty of company around me. The problem, of course, was that I lacked the basic knowledge and ability to plug into this source of company, especially when there was such a diverse group of people from all over the country there, and shared experiences and points of reference could not be assumed. As is my habit in any new environment, I developed a routine with which I felt familiar regarding shopping, laundry, study, and lectures, and within a couple of weeks I was more comfortable and felt able to put my initial disquiet down to going "cold turkey" away from the familiarity of what I had grown up with. After all, the wider world was what I had wanted to experience by moving away from that home environment and so I reasoned that this had been a necessary step to achieve that. And one could experience that from the side-lines if required.

The next problem with mixing in was that, although it was an all-male residence hall, I was in a University in the East Midlands, and guys from "the South" were not that common, or all that welcome it seemed. I had to get used to a different male company and environment to that which I was used to, as well as having to deal with the universal antipathy towards anyone who hailed from south of the Watford Gap. This was not just related to my origin, but also my apparent unwillingness to drink far too much and vomit excessively on a regular basis. However, I did make a few friends. The hall of residence was a chimera of an old ivy-clad building with sash windows and appalling insulation, and a newer extension which had been built as a mirror image of the previous building and wings, so that the entirety formed a square enclosing a central quad with grass and pathways. My room was in the newer half, which lacked some of the architectural character but gained significantly in comfort and warmth, so I was happy enough there. The food was good and filling, if somewhat basic, and I had no complaints. I kept some biscuits and other comestibles in my room but found that one of my friends, who came round every evening to watch my small black and white television and snack at will, reduced the supplies considerably without ever contributing to them. Even when I just wanted an evening on my own, this friend would stand outside the door knocking on it until given entry having seen that my light was lit on the way over from his own room in an adjacent residence. It will come as no surprise to learn that I was not entirely sure how to confront him about this situation back then, and so it just continued.

My mother had prepared me well for a certain level of self-sufficiency by giving me various ad hoc lessons on elementary cooking, the rudiments of laundry and ironing, and basic financial budgeting. However well prepared I felt that I was in these subjects, I would have swapped all this for the inside track on understanding girls. Because of those reasons already listed, girls were a closed book to me, and having an older sister made the subject no clearer as the four-year age difference between us meant that I was viewed as the annoying and embarrassing little brother, and me and my sister may as well have inhabited different planets by the time I was a teenager myself. I had never so much as caught a girl's eye whilst walking down the street, and I did not even know that this was a thing. I had always just stared straight ahead with tunnel vision, and I still do much the same today when on my own. But that is when there are people about. On a walk in the countryside my gaze is everywhere, at the birds and other wildlife, the weather, the crops in the fields, and at any company with me, be it Suzy or the dogs, or both. Back then, if I had noticed anybody looking my way, I would certainly have looked the other way rather than return the gaze. My early tentative forays upon this foreign field of adult relationships were easily rebuffed leaving me hurt and confused, and so I retreated behind my usual defences, with occasional peeks from behind them being all that I dared. I could not readily make head nor tail of what I observed though. It seemed to me as if social life was actually a game to which everyone else knew the rules, and were considerably experienced with them, but were not prepared to share them with me. Phrases such as "Don't you know?" and "It is obvious isn't it?" were the incredulous answers to tentative questioning of my peers on the subject, and so I simply stopped asking and decided to avoid the situations instead. It seemed to me a bit like the idea that you need three people in the telling of a joke, one to tell it, another to laugh at it, and another who does not get it. The enjoyment of the first two is meant to be heightened by the fact that the third person clearly does not understand something that the others share and do get enjoyment from. What supporters of this theory seem to overlook is the potential misery and embarrassment of that third person, especially as the idea is not to explain the joke to them but laugh at the fact that they are not party to a shared understanding that the other two people have.

There were few people in whom I would even confide this lack of awareness, and I was somewhat hesitant to do this given my natural reticence, and the failure of those confidants I did have to help me out meant that I just retreated from the embarrassment and confusion of those situations. My best friend at university seemed to have had plenty of previous experience before arriving and continued in much the same vein once there, easily accomplishing liaisons with female students studying there or even just visiting. Whilst he seemed to be able to just help himself at will to the smorgasbord of opportunity all around him, I felt as if I was at a table for one in the corner without even a menu to guide me, and just watching whilst others made the best of their youthful confidence.

I had a couple of short-lived relationships and neither of them had a sexual element. One girl, a colleague on my course, was on the rebound from a long-term relationship and, although things seemed to have been going well to me, she called a halt fairly early on. I, of course, said I understood her reasoning for this completely and I allowed her the freedom and breathing space she yearned for, and from which she promptly escaped with somebody other than me. I could not understand why she had not contacted me when she felt the time was right as she had implied that she would, and at which word I had taken her. Clearly it was me that she did not want, rather than managing a new relationship so soon after the previous one had broken down. There was another girl that I went out with a couple of times, and I then invited her along to the annual party at my hall of residence, splashing out on a ticket for her. She seemed pleased to be invited and we entered the party fray together, but by the time I had fought my way to the bar and returned with drinks for us both, she had disappeared. I failed to find her for most of the evening, even missing the band that was playing in doing so. This was a new band that nobody had heard of at the time but was playing small gigs like university bars – they were called Culture Club. You may have heard of them. I eventually found my date dancing with somebody else and saying that she felt no obligation to remain in my company all evening just because I had purchased her ticket. Whilst implying no ownership as such, I had felt that a date implied that one would stay together for the course of that evening, or at least explain the situation if that proved too much to bear, rather than just taking oneself off to find entertainment elsewhere. Was nothing as it seemed? I never tried the hall party again.

By the end of my five-year course, I had still learnt little of the dark arts of dating and that shadowy world at the end of the evening when the disco had ended or the pub had turned out, when I never really knew what was going to happen or why and

I seemed to be able to exert no influence on it anyway.

The other thing that was part of my personality was that I tended to take things at face value: in other words, I did not play games in relationships or anything else, and did not understand others that did, either in their motivation or their meaning. Therefore, if a girl said they did not want to see me, I took it that this is what they meant. Being told later that this was only said to make me keener to be in touch, the idea that you would want something even more if it had been withheld, simply did not make sense to me, and smacked of manipulation. I did not realise that this was all part of the courtship in those that understood the game. I dealt more in the black and white of a situation and so felt you should say exactly what you meant and then you both knew where you stood.

One thing that I was certain of was that I hated night clubs. I did not enjoy them and could not see the point of them. They were expensive, especially for a student as discounted entry on certain nights for students were not common then. However, one still had to run the gauntlet of the bouncers to see if they deigned to let you in so that you could part company with your money. The clubs were incredibly noisy, to such an extent that I found the volume overwhelming and the crush of people around me unsettling. I also found myself deaf for quite some time upon escaping back out into the city centre. I went twice in the five years I was there. The second time was to see if it really was as bad as I thought it had been the first time. It was, despite so many people saying how great the club atmosphere was. Also, before the ban on smoking in enclosed public places, clubs were full of smoke which set me coughing and my eyes smarting. It also meant that every single item of clothing smelt of smoke afterwards, right down to the underwear. Pubs were no better in this regard, although at least one could escape to the beer garden outside in the summer months. My reaction to the club environment was probably why I also disliked firework displays. All that jostling in a crowd in the dark, followed by a visual and auditory assault, and the visceral thump of the loud explosions.

I tolerated a few for the sake of my children when they were younger, but I have never liked them nor felt comfortable in that environment.

I did enjoy both university and medical school despite all of the difficulties outlined above. Firstly, the city was a good place to be a student, being compact and accessible, and having a university, polytechnic college (which has since become another university), radiography school, nursing school, and physiotherapy school so plenty of young adults around and the place felt as if it had a youthful vibe, even if I did not fully participate in that. The university hospital was brand new. So brand new, in fact, that it was not fully opened at the time of my studying there and was still not completely in use when I left after five years. I spent my clinical training trying to find various parts of the new hospital and occasionally running into locked wards with equipment and no staff, or corridors festooned with polythene sheets as fittings were completed. There was also a much older hospital on the other side of town which the medical students also attended for clinical experience. However, this one still had the old nightingale style wards, with rows of beds along each wall and only curtains to partition them rather than bays so that anything that happened to one patient was audible to the rest of the ward. There were also ancient, tiled corridors and covered outdoor walkways and mysterious corridors and flights of stairs leading to who knows where.

The medical school was separated from the university campus by a fearfully busy ring road that would have been impassable without the pedestrian bridge that crossed it and led from just outside the main entrance to the outskirts of the campus. The bridge was enclosed and smelled strongly of rubber from the textured flooring it had, whose pungent aroma did not seem to diminish with the passage of time or the thousands of feet which tramped its length daily. The bridge led to the main campus which was large and picturesque with wide open grassed areas, plenty of trees, and an undulating landscape within which the various halls of residence were thinly scattered. There was an adjacent park and lake, which was pressed into service for many adventurous competitions, especially in and around Fresher's Week, and a back entrance which led to a gate in the high wall of an adjacent mansion, a former stately home, which had its own delightful parkland. Although I was only resident on campus for two years, I made regular visits back to the campus for various reasons, and I never tired of it. Having graduated, I went back only once, some ten years after leaving the University, and found, to my relief and gratification, that it had retained its charm.

Those first two years when I lived in the campus hall accommodation were part of the three pre-clinical years of training, when most of the work of the course was undertaken in lecture theatres, laboratories, and the anatomy suite where human bodies were dissected to better inform the three-dimensional aspects of human anatomy, as opposed to the two-dimensional representations in the textbooks. Having overcome my initial horror of this task, I found it immensely absorbing to discover just how everything went together, as well as the enormous number of variations from the basic human blueprint that were possible and considered normal. The final two years were more clinically based and depended upon the attendance at ward rounds and watching or helping in operating theatres, as well as stints on delivery floor and in casualty, intended to give a rounded view of the profession but invariably meaning that the student got an extremely limited view via the tasks that nobody else wanted to do. Experience in Accident and Emergency, for example, was much less about witnessing major trauma or life-saving interventions, and much more about stitching up an ever-increasing list of people with minor skin lacerations who would otherwise have to be attended to by the Senior House Officer under whose tutelage the students were meant to be for that shift. This helped develop my skill in suturing but did little to broaden my medical knowledge or experience. Similarly, on the delivery floor there were midwifery students who had to witness a specific number of births as part of their training. As medical students did not have this requirement we were always last in the queue to witness them, and I then did not see any more until I was suddenly in charge of them as a junior doctor.

Another example of this was during a surgical attachment when a patient was admitted onto the ward with a leaking aneurysm of his abdominal aorta. This dilation of a weak point in the main artery taking blood from the left side of the heart, is similar to a blow-out in a bicycle tyre inner tube where the pressure within can no longer be controlled by the strength of the tube wall. It can lead to catastrophic internal haemorrhage and rapid demise, but in some cases the pressure of the tissues surrounding the leak help to stem the flow so that rapid repair of the artery can save the patient's life. The surgical team needed an extra pair of hands, and I was chosen. I have no recollection of volunteering for this, and I can only presume that I failed to take the requisite backwards step in time. I had the apparently vital job of looking after the mass on intestines, whose attachment to the posterior abdominal wall had been severed to allow access to the aorta, and they had been put into a large plastic bag for me to watch over until they could be reattached. I was to tell the surgeon if the intestines looked at all blue as their blood supply also came off the aorta and such a change in appearance could indicate that their circulation had become compromised.

The surgery was being done by a Senior Registrar, his first such operation, and supervised by the consultant, and it took well over seven hours, starting at around eight in the evening. It was hard to remain alert over that length of time, standing stock still on hard wooden clogs on a hard tiled floor at the side of the operating table, whilst the two surgeons discussed the minutiae of each suture involving the damaged aorta and the graft that they were repairing it with, like two members of an overly fastidious crochet circle. It was seven hours of mind-numbing, back-breaking, feet-screaming tedium, relieved only partially by taking my feet out alternately from their clogs and placing them against the deliciously cool metal base of the operating table for a bit of respite from the sustained pressure on them. All the time I was watching the intestines like a hawk for any hint of a violaceous hue, whilst peristalsis made them writhe in a languid and soporific manner, like a post-prandial python, the visual equivalent of white noise. I was also ravenously hungry. I had always found that helping at surgical operations made my saliva run and my stomach growl, to the extent that I began to wonder whether my family tree had some Transylvanian branch hidden in the mists of time that nobody talked about, but it seems that this is just a physiological response and could normally be appeased by the consumption of something before entering the operating theatre. Unfortunately, I had not had that opportunity on this occasion.

When the operation was at last over, the two surgeons repaired to the rest room for celebratory coffee and sandwiches which had been conjured for them by the theatre sister. I was dismissed at a flick, like a bogey from a finger, from there to get changed and walk home alone, through dank and deserted streets, back to my shared flat where the fridge was as empty as a politician's promise.

During those first two years, I did get a little non-medical real-life experience via a summer job that I took. After that, the lengthening terms of the medical course meant that I never again got a long summer vacation. The job I had was as a computer operator at a company that dealt with seismic exploration for oil reserves. The crucial thing was that I did not need to know anything about computers which was fortunate as I did not. Computers at that stage were still on the largeish side so that a bank of them that fitted snugly inside a fair-sized room had a similar power to your modern smart television. My job was to take a flow sheet from the programming department and follow it. There were various stock tapes that were the starting point for each of these flow sheets and each were about the size and weight of a metal dustbin lid. I had to load them onto the front of a computer, start the tape and then shut the front door to form a vacuum whereby the tape was sucked into a portal and the drum would start to rotate. Then a programme would be fed into a slot by means of a deck of cards with various ranks of square punched holes along their length. The intake would suck them in rapidly and then spit them out into a pile at the other end. The computer would then download the amalgamation of tape and programme onto another tape which would then need to be loaded and have another deck of cards fed in as the next step on the flow chart, and so on until the resulting end tape had to be labelled and put onto a rack for collection. It was mind-numbingly boring with the only light relief being if one of the cards was slightly bent and would not go in the feed slot but would hover in the suction like a broomstick waiting for the off in quidditch, and the card would have to be retrieved, straightened, and presented back to the slot. The job was worked in 12-hour shifts, four days on, four days off, four nights on, four days off and so on. At least the pay was reasonable and a welcome boost, but the working environment was not all it could have been. Even in the toilets, the cubicle walls were coated with a layer of dried bogeys where the users had picked their nose whilst at their ablutions and then wiped the resulting finger-load onto the walls. At least it covered up some of the graffiti. Two summers of working there was more than enough, and the idea of a career in such an environment did not bear thinking about.

After my two years of living in hall, I was obliged to move out into rented accommodation within the city for the remainder of the course, and so I followed the usual pattern of starting with the dregs left by those experienced students who sorted their accommodation out early, and then slowly improving my living quarters in following years by experience and gradually getting in earlier, eventually managing to take over the better accommodation as senior students graduated and left their flats vacant. As mentioned, it was usual for students moving out for the first time to leave it too late and find that all the best properties had been let for the following year. Therefore, the first house that I shared with three other students on my course was dire. It was on a corner busy with traffic heading into and out of the city, such that any open window let in dirt and noise, but the house was so cold that opening any window was a bad idea anyway. Having said that, I several times noted that the house interior seemed to be colder than the prevailing outdoor temperature and so an open window might have helped. There were gaps under all the doors, no doubt so that the mice did not have to crouch too much to get in and out, and the only heating available was from expensive and ineffective convector heaters. The only hot water came from an immersion heater that was also hideously expensive to use. Us flatmates therefore used to shower in the gym facilities after any sports activities, or otherwise at the medical school in showers that were intended for use by medics who had been working in theatres, but which were always seemingly full of students. In the house, we used the kettle to heat enough water to wash up dishes or to shave in and went as long as possible between these episodes without going as far as growing a beard. This was fortunate as several of the property owners of better accommodation refused to let their flats out to students with beards, apparently believing that wearing facial hair equated to moral turpitude. So, we learned from our initial mistakes and arranged much more comfortable, quiet, and clean accommodation for the remaining two years of our studies. This was in an area called The Park, which was made up of large, well-proportioned houses of faded grandeur, the former residences of merchants or other well-to-do citizens, but now divided into apartments and mostly inhabited by students. The roads were wide and undulating as the area spanned a distance from the top of the escarpment overlooking the city, down to the river that ran beside it. The area was closer to the city than the medical school and so allowed a certain separation between work and leisure that the campus had not afforded.

One other thing that happened at university was that I suffered from depression. This was mild, I realised when looking back later, and was never treated, but it still descended like a suffocating cloak for no apparent reason and hung around for days or weeks. Once there, it stupefied thought and left me just wanting to be alone. I withdrew to my room and either just sat in misery or listened to mournful music. It affected my motivation to do anything, and the ability to concentrate if I tried to do anything. I sought no help for this, indeed I never considered doing so, for I did not understand it at the time. My best friend definitely did not understand, bemoaning my isolation as self-indulgence and encouraging me to "just bloody cheer up," a form of words reminiscent to me of those used by Basil Fawlty when he was exhorting Manuel to get himself out of the doldrums, and just as unlikely to succeed. Of course, this cheering up of myself lay outside my power at the time, and I just hung in there, knowing from experience that it would pass. Later in practice, I realised just how many young adults face mental health issues, and how many of them were considerably more serious than that which I had faced. I was always able to get through my episodes when they occurred, but many more found themselves unable to function or cope with daily activities for long periods at a time and found that the mood of melancholy would pervade all aspects of their life, both emotional and physical. Part of the difficulty of diagnosing at times is that there is the phenomenon of somatisation, whereby emotional anguish manifests as physical symptoms. However, my experience gave me insight into how someone might be feeling with depression, even if there was a difference in the degree of severity, and so it informed how I dealt with these patients. I realised that I was lucky that it passed after a few years without recourse to medication, and that many were not so lucky. I was also pleased for the patient population of the UK that once my friend had qualified he subsequently went into a specialism that did not primarily involve engaging with patients' mental health.

Later in my career I taught consulting skills on post-graduate modules for health care professionals at the local university's School of Health Sciences. One of the exercises that I got students to do was to work in pairs, and I gave one of the pair a picture that was a pattern made up of different shapes. The task was for that student to describe the pattern to their partner, who could not see it but whose task it was to replicate it on a plain piece of paper. Their partner could ask as many questions as they liked, and they were allowed 10-15 minutes to complete the task, at the end of which they compared their pattern to the original to see how close their effort was. The results were usually broadly similar and depended upon the describing skills of one student, and the listening and interpretative skills of the other. I would then ask the group what they thought the point of the exercise was. The answers were usually along the lines of demonstrating effective communication. I would then ask them how they got so close to the original, and the responses were less clear but normally included elements such as the use of language and having similar terms of reference for elements such as shape and position. The next step would be to then ask the students to consider how they would go about the same task if there was no pattern but instead somebody had to describe their pain, or their mood, and consider how easy that was to do, especially when one could not make a direct comparison at the end of the task to see how close their effort was. If terms of reference were not shared, and if powers of description were not good, the impression gained could be a long way from the actual detail being described.

This was also the basis of the somatisation mentioned earlier, where patients may find symptoms impossible to describe except in physical terms. For instance, the sensation of anguish might well be best described by the lay person as "pain." I would ask the students to consider this aspect when they next took a history. This exercise also showed how one could draw from one's own life experience to get a sense of what the patient was trying to get across, and this would help the doctor to empathize with them. However, I took pains to point out that context was significant and that remarkably similar sounding symptoms could have a vastly different impact on one person from another, depending upon what else was going on with that person, and thus they should be careful not to confuse "I can see how difficult that must be for you" with "I know how you feel." The terms of reference may be made clearer by a similar experience, but they were likely to remain different and this should always be borne in mind.

I remained consistent in my manner and habits. Although I had been exposed to punk and ska at school, and the New Romantic movement, reggae, and other more esoteric genres at university subsequently, I took tracks that I liked from these and was never completely won over by any of them, and certainly would never have considered becoming part of a sub-culture. Perhaps I was already a sub-culture compared to those round me. I had developed a liking for rock music in the 1970s, and this grew and has remained for the rest of my life, though I never went as far as going to gigs or wearing tour t-shirts or long hair. I cherry-picked the elements that appealed and discarded the rest and one could never tell my preferences from without. Indeed, several people were surprised by my choice of music. For some reason I felt duty bound to delve into opera and classical music, although I could not have said why other than with an element of experimentation. It had never been played at home, although Dad liked a bit of Mario Lanza, and I was not keen on that. It always seemed to me that classical music equated to culture and that one was supposed to like it as culture was linked to education. Although I liked some of it, the genre held no on-going appeal and it never spoke to me the way a guitar riff or solo did, and thus rock remained my first love. I can accept that others become just as absorbed in a soaring aria as I do in a guitar solo, but I also know that generally such music is not for me. Much of it I found physically painful to endure. It was problematic that nobody I was close to shared my preference for rock music, and thus I became used to my music choices being labelled simply as "that noise."

I have always viewed musical appreciation, and the appreciation of other things such as art and beauty, like simple harmonic motion. Any music heard would influence the person hearing it, either in a positive or negative way, but there was often one genre or musical phrasing that hit exactly the right point, that chimed with something within, such that the resultant resonance was much exaggerated and the response to it was much greater. This is what I felt with the rock music, though I could never hope to emulate it. I managed to teach myself to the point that I could strum a bit on the guitar, but I never took playing more seriously than that, and I was not committed to it. I could not read music and felt that this went along with my poor ability with languages, for what was music if not another language with units, flow, inflection, and moods of its own. I also liked acoustic ballads, despite them being at the other end of the scale of popular music, and so my tastes as a playlist made an eclectic mix at times, although rock still had a playlist to itself.

Despite my social ineptitude, I made a small group of friends whilst at university. However, I tended to be the one to compromise on any given subject or activity to avoid conflict and argument, and eventually with my initial best friend, who was also a medical student, my own choices and preferences were being subtly usurped. We always ended up doing what this friend wanted, whilst he, my friend, always belittled anything that I expressed a liking or preference for. This seemed to be one of the reasons why I lost confidence in my own choices over time and tended to submit to those of others. After three years of this pattern, I had had enough and we parted company, both as housemates and companions, but I remained vulnerable to this subtle act of manipulation and was the victim of it several times throughout my life, including in my first marriage. Whether I was particularly vulnerable, and this was recognised by the other parties, or whether they were just particularly good at it, I never really decided, but, for some reason, I repeatedly failed to spot the pattern and only recognised it in retrospect.

One of the things that helped in the later clinical years at university was having a car. I was quite a late learner regarding driving, having not passed my test until I was twenty-one, but I had received a small legacy following the death of an aged relative and used this to purchase my pride and joy, a gold-coloured Ford Escort Mark two 1300E. It had a walnut veneer fascia overlay, a vinyl roof, and the coveted Rostyle wheels. This helped with getting around to the various clinical attachments I had, and the University clearly expected some of the students to have cars as attendance at some of the furthest establishments would have been impossible using public transport alone. I kept the car for several years but never forgot the sense of freedom that I had gained by its acquisition, even though I had to fit lockable wheel nuts and deadbolts to the doors after several break-ins. Well, not so much break-ins but the locks on early Fords were so poor that it was said you could gain entry by using a wet kipper as a key and it would still work. I also realised that I had to nurture the car as it did not feel like it wanted to go too fast on long trips, such as those between home and The Midlands. I would always break the journey at Cambridge and spend a pleasant hour wandering around this city before driving on in whichever direction I was going, the Escort always seeming to be grateful for the breather and running better on the second leg of the journey. It was at the time when all cars, though much simpler mechanically than those of today, also seemed to have their own foibles and personality. I had to do things in a certain order to encourage it to start. The right procedure always worked, but if a start was attempted without two pulses on the accelerator with full choke, followed by pushing the choke halfway back and swiftly turning the key, then it would not start, and I would have to sit and wait for five minutes before trying it again with the correct procedure.

CHAPTER 6

One thing that I did do, once freed by the university environment from what I saw as my self-imposed restrictions on behaviour at home, was to be a little more adventurous, although this seemed in retrospect to be contrary to most of my personality traits. I was never going to be one who went dramatically off the rails or breached new frontiers, but there were two things that I achieved and was pleased with.

The first was making a parachute jump. I had never been particularly good with heights, and I hated any kind of fairground ride. I had even felt physically sick on playground swings as a child. I had never understood how other children could swing so wildly and with evident delight, whereas I just felt ill and disliked the forwards movements, though found the reverse swing a little more tolerable. This was quite apart from the fact that the swings would be sited on a hardstanding back then rather than the cushioned play surfaces of modern times, and any fall was likely to have had profound consequences. Once older and medically qualified I realised that I had a sensitive vestibular apparatus in my inner ear and therefore was intolerant of rapid or rapidly changing movements, but at the time I just felt like a wimp and so avoided such supposed amusements. Even when I was older, fairground rides and theme parks held no attraction for me. The idea of paying excessively for the opportunity to join a long queue, and then wait half an hour or so just to for a chance to feel physically sick, made no sense to me at all. Not surprisingly, this further pragmatic approach to stark reality tended to add to my label of being no fun to have around. Again, there was this pressure to conform, usually phrased along the lines of "Why can't you just join in and have some fun?" The idea that it might not be fun for me to join in never seemed to occur to others, and many people simply have no idea that not everybody experiences life or the world around them in the same way that they do and thus it does not occur to them to make allowance for this.

Once at university I had found that there was both a former friend of mine from our Primary school days, and a good school friend of my brother, both on the same campus as me and both studying Civil Engineering. I mixed with that group of lads a bit and found that they had arranged to do a static-line parachute jump, for no particular reason other than they just fancied it, and they asked if I wanted to join them. Despite this conversation being over a pint or two, which always oiled the wheels of cooperation a bit, nobody was more surprised than I was when I said "Yes," and so it was arranged. This surprise was because I was anything but spontaneous. One of the things that marked my personality was that I felt comfortable with a routine once I had established one. It gave me comfort and the impression that I had some control over things. I had established one to get comfortable with being at university in the first place, with the structure of lectures in the week, shopping on a Saturday, laundry on a Sunday etc. so for me to have just agreed to anything as outrageous as a parachute jump, on a whim, was certainly out of character for me. Once having made the commitment, I was determined not to back out, but felt it best not to mention anything to my parents about the plan beforehand in case they worried or tried to persuade me not to. Instead, I decided it would be better just to ring afterwards with my opening phrase being "Guess what I was doing today."

The group of us duly turned up at the local airstrip on what had turned out to be a glorious day in mid-October during my second year of the medical course, with bright sunshine showing off the clear blue of the vast sky with the occasional fluffy cloud passing by. We spent the morning in training with the instructor and aimed to make a jump in the afternoon. We started with details of the day's itinerary, lectures on wind speed and drop velocity, explanation and demonstrations of the equipment involved, the inevitable health and safety concerns and how they were to be addressed, communication signals once airborne, and much more. There then came the exercises which consisted of lying on the ground and adopting the arched body position that would be required once out of the aircraft and dropping like a stone and ended in jumping off a ramp to do the appropriate landing from height. This required us keeping our knees tucked tight together and semi-flexed, landing with both feet together, and then rolling so that the point of impact travelled from the feet up the side of one leg and then the side of the body so that the shock of landing at speed was thus dissipated rather than there being a sudden deceleration which could break a bone. There was also the exercise of wearing a harness suspended from the ceiling and then going through drills for finding tangled straps on the parachute once deployed, having a damaged parachute, the deploy of the reserve chute, and other things that we all earnestly hoped would not be needed. That last drill, to deploy the reserve chute if the main one failed to open, whilst plummeting towards earth at a speed that made the height of the jump seem entirely inadequate, seemed particularly concerning. The entire day was fuelled by adrenaline, bravado, coffee, and large numbers of filled rolls, or "cobs" as they were called in this part of England, from the cafeteria on site. When our instructors were satisfied with our standard, by which time it was mid-afternoon, we were given the all-clear to go up and perform the jump.

This was a significant thing for I had never flown before, which was one of the reasons that I had surprised myself by agreeing to join the day. Our family had never taken holidays abroad as we could not afford to do so, and so I had never travelled higher up than the front seat on the top deck of the number 94 bus to Bromley. And now here I was, kitted out in a jumpsuit and parachute pack, with helmet and goggles, walking uncertainly and in an ungainly fashion across the runway towards our aircraft. This was not just due to anticipation of what was to come, but because the straps of the harness cut into my thighs, and I found myself adopting something of the gait I had seen all too often on cowboys from old Westerns. Once I had got to our destination, I was looking at what appeared to be a toy aircraft that was half missing. It was, in fact, a Cessner with a single propeller on the nose, wings that sat across the top of the flight cabin, and half the side missing from behind where the pilot sat. I thought that it looked very insubstantial and that the chances of me jumping were only slightly greater than the chances of me falling out before we got to the right place. But I was determined to see it through and so, somewhat awkwardly, I managed to clamber on board with my friends. We had to climb in backwards and then shuffle across the cabin floor to sit between each other's legs for the duration of the flight, as if we were going to sing along to "Oops upside your head." Once we were at the correct height and conditions were acceptable, and only when told to do so by the jump manager, we would then have to shuffle forward to the open side of the aircraft, one after the other, and sit with our legs hanging out over the sill and into the slipstream, having previously clipped our rip cord to an anchorage on the fuselage. We were to do a static line jump from two and a half thousand feet, so there was no free fall involved. With the parachute release secured to the aircraft, once we had slipped over the side and started the rapid drop, our body weight would deploy the parachute as we plummeted earthwards, and it should be fully deployed after we had travelled for a count of ten seconds. We should have been counting off those seconds and then at that point our descent would be suddenly arrested by the parachute opening and we could look up to check the situation regarding our lines and the state of the canopy. If there was no sudden jerk at ten seconds, then we should go into the drill to deploy our reserve. That, at least, was the theory.

The aircraft had bumped and rattled its ponderous way across to the runway and, having then accelerated noisily and uncomfortably over the grass, it tilted its nose upwards alarmingly and started its ascent. I could then see why the hand signals were so useful as I could not hear anything above the sound of the engine and the wind as it whipped past the open fuselage. We were to jump at a point over the airstrip and aim to land within a circle some twenty yards across. We were to use the windsocks on the airstrip to try to gauge the wind and thus adjust during our drop. Vents in the rear of the canopy directed air flow as we dropped and allowed some directional control and pulling on one side of the harness or the other allowed us to turn so that we were facing the way we wished to go and the airflow from the vents propelled us in that direction, always taking the direction of the prevailing wind into account and allowing for it. To avoid over-running the target area as we got closer to it, we could aim in a rough circle as we dropped by manoeuvring the harness straps.

As we got nearer the jump point the instructor looked at me with some concern and I realised I must have gone as white as sheet. I was certainly regretting some of those rolls, but I was determined to complete my chosen task, and so I shuffled over to sit on the edge of the plane when my turn came. I attached the ripcord to the fuselage point and twisted to the side to sit on one buttock, and looked upwards towards the underside of the wing, as instructed, and then let myself off the side when given the all-clear by a touch on the shoulder. Now obviously I had just jumped out of a plane at over two thousand feet, but for some reason I was not prepared for the sensation that followed as I dropped like a stone earthwards. Whenever I had seen parachutists on the television, they were always filmed from somebody who had jumped with them and who was therefore dropping at the same rate as them. Compared to a fixed point I was dropping away at the rate of a speeding car and I was just not prepared for how disorientating it felt. It was a good learning experience for me to find that no matter how much training you do, nothing can prepare you for the actual event, and that there was no substitute for having experienced something. It was a similar experience I would later have when I stepped out onto the ward as a qualified doctor three years later knowing a substantial amount about anatomy, physiology, pathology, and pharmacology but having no idea about what the job itself entailed.

From the moment of my exit from the plane, as mentioned, I was meant to countdown to that time at which I should have been abruptly slowed by the opening of the parachute and I could look up to check the straps and canopy itself. However, the shock of my sudden and rapid descent was such that this countdown awareness was lost almost immediately. I felt the sudden lurch and deceleration as my parachute canopy opened, and at least I had the wherewithal to look up and check the kit. However, on the way down I realised that I would never have been in a fit state to have counted and deployed my reserve if that had been needed. Therefore, it might as well not have been there and so, long before I reached the ground, I had made the firm resolve never to do that again. It was not a decision I ever regretted. However, since I was up there, I did make the most of the fabulous view, with the sun slowly sinking towards the western horizon and seeming to set the few straggling clouds ablaze. I landed roughly where intended, with little more than a sore elbow because of not tucking it in properly as I rolled on landing. I stood and collected my parachute up in my arms by walking towards it into the wind and spooling it on my arms, and then carried it back to base. We were all elated by our successful day. Fortunately, nobody had got injured beyond the odd bump or graze, and we travelled back to university in high spirits, where a few congratulatory pints were sunk. The day's events were told and re-told, and gradually elements of the day became augmented in much the same way as anglers relate the size of the fish that got away. A bond had been formed that lasted the rest of the time at university but, unfortunately, not the parting of the ways thereafter as the group members were scattered to diverse parts of the British Isles, and work responsibilities claimed most of our attention.

I had to wait until the end of my course for the other main adventure, which was a trip to Australia, but it was well worth it. Like so many British medical courses, the one that I was on had a six-week period timetabled at the end of the final year during which the students were allowed to go anywhere they wished to gain experience in a field of medicine or surgery of their choice, or to see how health services functioned in other countries. This time was known as "the elective". The only catch was that the medical school's only input was to allow us the time in which to take this opportunity, and the students had to arrange and fund the whole thing themselves. As with medical students elsewhere, my cohort was scattered all over the globe because of this opportunity. Some sought out experience in specialist fields at home, often with an eye on improving their Curriculum Vitae ahead of an intended specialism to forge a career in, whilst others travelled abroad to experience both healthcare systems and life more generally, in another country. Members of my cohort went to the Americas, the West Indies, all parts of Europe, or, like me, to Australia. My own choice had been dictated by circumstance as much as anything, but I felt that, if I were to travel somewhere then I might as well do it properly and go as far as possible. This was partly because I had never flown abroad before, but also because I felt that I may not get the chance again any time soon, or ever.

I had been doing an attachment in Paediatrics as part of my undergraduate training, and I had been based for this at a hospital in another city in the same region of England, but too far to commute daily. Therefore, accommodation was found for students on placement in the nursing residence attached to that hospital. The potential problems with this arrangement, in the days when there were more male students than female ones and nursing was almost entirely a female preserve, seemed to have been overlooked by the medical school and the authorities of the nursing residence, and it was not an unpopular arrangement. I did try to capitalise on this opportunity, but it will come as no surprise that I did not make any progress in the two weeks that I was there beyond occasional group trips for a pint or two in the local pubs. However, as well as the resident nurses and other medical students in my attachment group, I met a visiting Australian student called, of all things, Bruce. He must have had a skin like a rhino to survive the ribbing he would have got in the UK where it was considered that Bruce was a generic name for anyone from Down Under, but he was easily capable of giving as good as he got and was thoroughly likeable. Anyway, I took the opportunity of asking him about his medical school in Australia and then cadging the name and address of the dean of that medical school from him. I then took a chance and wrote to the dean to ask if I could be accommodated to come to that medical school on my elective the following year. Fortunately, the answer was in the affirmative, and so I began to organise the trip.

The first obstacle to overcome was the cost of the ticket. Thirty-five years might have gone by since that time, but the cost of a return flight to Australia was greater back then than it is now, and I had to fund that somehow. I knew that it would be well beyond my parent's means, and I would not have asked them anyway after they had helped to fund my living expenses at university. Fortunately, I had been prudent throughout my university life and had budgeted as my mother had advised me to, so my account had never gone overdrawn. That gave me a good background for a loan with the bank that I used for the fare, and to obtain a credit card, a rare acquisition for my age back then, for backup funds so I did not get stuck for money once away in an unknown country with unknown costs and eventualities. I then researched the area I was going to, bearing in mind that there were no computers or internet back then to use to access such information. I read and used information from libraries and travel agents to augment the information that I had got from Bruce once I explained to him what my plans were. There were few specialist travel shops for backpacking or similar foreign trips for me to access information from at that time, and no publications for such adventures, and without today's communications technology there could be no websites, chatrooms, or social media platforms to use. The most adventurous that most students got was to travel around Europe over the summer using a railcard. I applied for a visa and received this just in time from the Australia High Commission after there was no sign of it as the date got close, and I had to write expressing the urgency of my request and the need for both the visa and my passport back.

At last, the final summer term had passed, I had completed my final year exams, and it was time to go on my trip whilst awaiting the results. My parents drove me across London to Heathrow airport, and I boarded the British Airways jumbo jet to Adelaide. This was a 24-hour long trip with two stops on the way, at Qatar and Singapore. There was much to negotiate on my own as I had never been in an airport before, and it was all new. I had been coached by colleagues who had travelled about the various steps of luggage weigh-in, passport control and security before accessing the departure lounge and having to look out for boarding information. I had still not had a holiday abroad in the time since my parachute jump, and so had not been up in an aircraft since. Also, although I had taken one flight in an aircraft, it was very much smaller, and I had never actually landed in one to know what that experience was like. However, I found the comfort and size of an airline seat vastly superior to the Cessner's cramped and juddering floor, and the food was reasonable. For all the circulating humour about the quality of airline food, I was, after-all, a student, and so could eat almost anything with evident relish. I was a little concerned about the possibility of a call going out during the flight that a doctor was needed for some medical emergency as, being a final year medical student, if there was no doctor about then I was probably the next best thing. Fortunately, this did not happen either way. Indeed, to date this has only happened once to me whilst flying somewhere, and it turned out to be something trivial anyway.

I got talking to a couple of fellow passengers en-route, and one of these was a Geordie ex-pat who now lived in Adelaide and was returning there from a visit to his family in the UK. This man kindly offered me a lift from the airport to the university campus in the foothills at the edge of the coastal plain on which the city of Adelaide sat, where I was to stay in university accommodation. As the man lived nearby, he also left his telephone number in case I failed to make friends once there and needed a friendly face to call upon or to meet up with.

The hospital and university were modern and set in a lovely, landscaped campus, with the sea in view in the middle distance, and good transport links to the city itself. The residence facilities were clean and modern, with a shared kitchen and bathroom, and so I was looking forward to my stay. I had a good-sized room with better general facilities than anything the NHS could boast within its own doctors' or nurses' quarters of my experience, which tended to be in Victorian wings with lofty ceilings and draughty windows.

Having settled in and walked around the hospital environs and nearby parts of the campus, I got something to eat and headed for an early night. I awoke the next day to the sound of unfamiliar birdsong. It was unfamiliar at the time anyway, as Australian dramas were not being screened on the television back home in the UK at that time. These days, however, the warbling birdsong, which sounds like a musical instrument clearing its throat, is much more familiar to British ears because of the popularity of such dramas. I got myself dressed, ready, and managed to find my way to the appropriate ward in the hospital where I was to gain further experience in Paediatrics and met up with the consultant in charge there and his team of junior doctors. I was assigned to one of the doctors on the team so that I could accompany him in his duties and spent the first day orientating myself around the relevant and vital parts of the hospital for my stay there, such as Accident & Emergency, the outpatients department, the paediatric wards, and the canteen. The latter was particularly important as fuel would be needed to keep me going.

It was interesting to find that the hospital was new to me and yet strangely familiar at the same time. There were some differences in nomenclature and protocols, but the actual business of assessing and treating sick children was broadly the same. The next day there was a ward round during which the whole team went around each patient under the care of the consultant, accompanied by a trolley which housed the patient's notes. Decisions were taken on the progress of treatment for each child, and these were written down prior to being acted upon. This entire process took an hour or two, after which I helped to clerk in the new admissions to the ward and observe their assessment and treatment. Clerking in a patient entails taking a full medical history and doing a relevant physical examination, and then documenting that in the patient record so that it could be easily seen and understood by anybody who was subsequently involved in the care of that patient.

The second day followed the same routine and on the third day, I came to the morning ward round again, only for the Senior Houseman I was accompanying to lean into me and say quietly "You know that you don't have to turn up *every* day, mate!" Clearly there was an understanding that part of the elective attendance was to immerse oneself in the local culture and not just the medical care of its population. Once it was made clear to me that this was both acceptable and to be encouraged, I subsequently took full advantage of the opportunity. Of course, there is always the chance that he just found it a giant pain in the neck having me tailing him around during his workday, but I like to think that he was just being kind.

I had already run into another medical student from the UK doing a similar thing to myself, in the same residence where I was staying and working in the same department. By coincidence, he had a younger sister at my own medical school and one of my flatmates apparently "had the hots" for this sister, which situation was a source of much amusement to my new colleague, Ash. He had come to this area of Australia to do his elective as he had friends who had emigrated there a few years earlier, and thus had local knowledge and companionship to engage with. I was invited to tag along with them and join in their outings and social life, and so tag along I did. It was early Autumn in the Southern hemisphere, but the days were still long, clear, and sunny, although the nights were getting cooler. Therefore, there were barbecues, trips to the beach, visits to wineries and their on-site restaurants, trips along the coast, the use of a friend's holiday home at Victor Harbour, and still the odd attendance at the hospital to be involved with the department and thus broaden my experience and justify the trip and the hospitality of the department that I was visiting. The one institution I discovered but could never see happening in the UK, was the drive-in off-license, or "offy" as it was known in the typical Australian short-hand for things. It implied a more liberal attitude to drinking and driving than I could envisage back home, where public safety campaigns were increasingly appearing in the media. Of course, time would show that some of these campaigns were fronted by personalities who, themselves, proved to be a different danger to the public, but nobody was aware of that at the time.

I loved the city of Adelaide, in whose outer suburbs the campus nestled. It was an attractive city with its broad expanse of low-rise suburbs stretching all the way to the sea from the Adelaide Hills. Out of this lagoon of bungalows, the high-rise city centre rose like the sheer cliffs of an island, the centre being separated from the outer by a perimeter of parkland which acted like the shore against which the sea of bungalows gently lapped but did not encroach. The city was clean, bright, and vibrant, with many distractions for the young and carefree. In these new surroundings, there was much to get used to – lager served in jugs with accompanying small schooner glasses, wine everywhere, food that included crayfish, abalone, and slipper lobsters (called "bugs" locally which made them sound a little less appetising), but also Vegemite spread and Tim-tam biscuits, Violet Crumble chocolate bars, and an open and friendly spirit. Other food stuffs on offer were more familiar, such as the meat pie upended in a lake of mushy peas, known as a "pie floater," and finished off by a generous application of ketchup. This was standard student fare in the East Midlands, but here it was bought from the pie carts that plied their wares at the roadside in Adelaide, especially after closing time for the bars and pubs. Surprisingly, some of my new Australian friends were aghast at my liking for it and thought it was an awful thing to eat. Whilst I found it delicious and welcome, I was a little perturbed by the fact that the pie contents were never defined any more specifically than as "meat." I did ask the provenance of the filling from one vendor, to be told that "As long as you find it tasty mate, it's probably best not to ask!"

I had never come across such an egalitarian lot as the Aussies, who would take you at face value and be glad to know you, notwithstanding a bit of ribbing, and they did not suffer fools gladly. Pomposity was not tolerated, and any inflated ego would soon be punctured by some barbed comment or another. Ian Botham's success in the recent Ashes series at the time certainly helped provide some retaliatory ammunition for me against "the colonials" and giving as good as you got was certainly an expectation, so generally an enjoyable time was had. There were, though, some elements similar to those back home, as a firm handshake and the ability to look somebody in the eye were taken as positive findings on first meeting, as was a lack of reticence about being the first at the bar, and these features helped towards being considered a "good bloke." That eye contact is an odd thing. Like many people with my condition, it can be a challenge. I would not seek to make eye contact with anybody in the street or a crowded room, indeed I studiously avoid doing so, but over the years I have managed to conquer the idea of doing so on first meeting somebody. Sustained eye contact is not so easy although it is an important part of trying to build rapport with a patient during a consultation, so I have had to learn to address that too. However, the Aussie trait of straightforwardness played to my strengths, and I never had to second guess what anybody meant when they said something. If they liked you or disliked you, agreed with you or didn't, then you knew about it immediately, and I much preferred it that way.

There was also much that sounded familiar. Here in Adelaide,

Brighton was close to Camden, and Dulwich and Hyde Park were not so far away. All the Glens added a Scottish note to the place names, but I discovered that they were named after the secretary of state at the time of the city's founding, rather than for those of the population who pledged their allegiance to the saltire.

One of the many new experiences for me was the wine as we were not a family of wine drinkers and so I had little experience of the gargle and spit variety. Of course, I was very well aware of the Monty Python sketch that was derogatory towards the whole idea of wines from Down Under, which were variously described by the comic team as having a kick like a mule, a lingering after-burn, and a bouquet like an aboriginal's armpit. Also, I knew little about wine in general as it was not something that was frequently drunk at university. My only experience was that a cheap way to get into a university party was to buy a bottle of hock at Sainsbury's for a pound or so, then hand it over on arrival and head for the cans of beer. Drinking it oneself was simply out of the question, regardless of how far gone one was. However, I accompanied my new friends on several trips to the Barossa Valley and the wineries there. These forays opened a world of wines to me, and the tasting sessions were informative and educational. There were red, rosé, and white, still and sparkling, cabernet sauvignon and chardonnay, as well as the wonderful restaurants that were also there to be sampled as part of the winery experience. It started an appreciation of good wine and food that has stayed with me thereafter, and which I cultivated and developed at some expense but much enjoyment.

I developed a liking for one girl in the group, an elfin extrovert who was noisy and popular, and thus was the polar opposite of myself. Whilst I was usually bookish and quiet, she would neck drinks and enter wet t-shirt competitions, and would take the mickey out of me whenever possible. Whilst our group were downing cocktails in the city one evening and I was emboldened with a couple of martinis inside me, I suggested to her that we share the strawberry garnish from her drink by holding it between my front teeth and inviting her to take half from me, which led to a kiss which we both seemed pleasantly surprised at. We then went out the following evening but after a couple of dates, I found myself being kept at arm's length, albeit done nicely, and she told me that she could not afford to fall for me as I was going soon and there was no future to it. Whilst upset at this, I was, once again, entirely understanding of her position and explanation. It was really the first time that I had considered that I might hold some attraction to a member of the opposite sex, and the idea that somebody might "fall" for me was a new revelation and offered some compensation for the disappointment that I felt. However, this was also the first time that I had acted with the reckless impetuosity that I had seen others undertake, and it did not help that I was rebuffed. It did profoundly knock my confidence to have tried and failed. If I had been able to ride that wave of burgeoning self-confidence, then who knows where it might have led. Instead, the surge dissipated and declined, never to return. The next impetuous thing that I did in my life was to ask Suzy, my second wife, out for a date some twenty-five years later. It was not the girl's fault, of course, as she only did what was right for her at the time and her reasoning was eminently sensible. However, she was also of a resilient type who would herself bounce back from any such setback immediately and would presumably expect others to as well. She was not to know that this did not apply to me and that by stepping on this early bloom of confidence she would crush it. But then that is true of us all, for we tend to judge others around us by our own standards and make little allowance for the possibility that others do not share the same psyche and outlook as ourselves. I have continued to accept compliments when they were offered but I have never whole-heartedly believed them. However, criticism would often leave me crushed.

In the last week of my time in Adelaide, I used my credit card to hire a small hatchback car and motored along the coast to see some of the natural beauty, as well as venturing into the Adelaide hills where recent wildfires from the summer had left their mark as darkened scars amongst the green canopy. I also admired some of the work-wear clothing I had seen on the locals and discovered that it was made in a small town on the outskirts of Adelaide so took a trip there. Here I bought some moleskin jeans, and stockman boots and was incredibly pleased with them. Though the boots eventually wore out after some twenty years, I replaced them, and a similar pair are still an item in my wardrobe all these years later. The moleskin jeans proved just as robust, though I tend to use them to walk the dogs in as they are hard wearing and comfortable, keeping most weather out other than heavy rain.

The six weeks of my stay passed all too quickly, and I soon found myself having to take my leave of this relative paradise to return home. On the long flight back to Heathrow, England, and home I reflected upon how I had gained more life experience in those few short weeks away from the usual and familiar than I had gained over the previous twenty-odd years in my natural environment. Of course, gap years, backpacking and trips "Down Under" are an obligatory rite of passage for the late teens and twenty-somethings of today, but such long-distance travelling was much less in evidence back then. Indeed, I remembered one of the medical professors at university giving a lecture about infectious diseases caught whilst abroad, and how travellers would venture off to the Indian subcontinent or elsewhere seeking experience and enlightenment and come back as "wrecks of humanity" having been ravaged by some unpleasant condition or another which lurked in the water, food, or insect life to snare the unwary. In my first week in Adelaide, I had been invited to go and camp in the bush by the doctor who had advised me not to turn up daily and who was spending a weekend away with some mates. I was appreciative of the offer but erred on the side of caution, feeling unprepared for that terrain and being uncertain of the company, but it was a decision that I regretted for ever afterwards. I vowed to return to the country that I had seen so little of but had come to think so much of, though that vow, to date, has not been realised.

Between the parachute jump and the elective trip, I felt that I had covered the two extremes of air travel at that point and so was certainly much more comfortable with it all on family holidays once my own children were born. That sort of air travel, though, brought all sorts of other challenges.

CHAPTER 7

Apart from medicine, the only other thing that I took with me from my time at university, was an enjoyment of running. I had never even considered doing that before, but I had been inspired by watching the inaugural London Marathon on the television during my first year of study at university, and so I took it up and found I enjoyed it. At first, I just used some ordinary trainers to run in, but found they did not support my feet adequately and caused them to ache, and there was no real cushioning of impact. I developed shin splints, a painful condition of the shins caused by repetitive impact trauma, and that led to some even more painful physiotherapy where scar tissue had to be broken down by hard manual massage, followed by the use of an ultrasonic device during healing, which was fortunately painless. The physio advised me to get some proper footwear if I was intent on continuing to run. I did some research into the subject via magazines and sports shops as there was still no internet to browse, and I found some Brooks running shoes going cheap in a sports shop because one of the pair had been in the window display and so had become faded by the sun. The change of footwear made all the difference, and it helped that I was on a campus university with parkland and open space nearby to run in. I was never going to win prizes, but that was not why I did it and, as with everything, I brought my own perspective to it. It was the perfect form of exercise for someone who preferred to undertake such activities alone. I had started go to the campus gym to use weights, but I disliked the competitive element to the atmosphere there. As with following the rules in team sports, if there was a particular way to lift a weight and do an exercise then that was the technique I followed. I could not be doing with those who used cheat lifting techniques to allow them to do more repetitions and then brag about the fact and look down on those of us who were not built like the proverbial brick out-house. Some people seem to want to turn everything in life into a competition. I bought some weights and a barbell and used them in my room thereafter. However, as well as the strengthening exercises, I wanted to do some cardiovascular activity. I had always enjoyed walking, but I found that a man out walking alone, without a dog or other obvious reason to be there, tended to be viewed with suspicion by any individual or group of women who happened to be walking in the same direction, and it was uncomfortable to keep having them cast cautious looks in my direction. Running fitted the bill nicely there as there could be no doubt at all what you were doing. Although I liked the running, I did not want any element of competition with other runners, I just wanted to do the run. It was me against the terrain and distance for that day. I did not worry about the weather. In fact, I enjoyed the added challenge of the elements and could not see the appeal of treadmills where you got nowhere and saw nothing and had to breathe stale moist air or else chill in air-conditioned surroundings. Also, treadmills could not mimic the changing terrain of the town, park, and countryside around me. Neither did I see the point in headphones and personal hi-fis, preferring to be in the moment of the run rather than have any distraction. I did not want to bother with personal best times, or training schedules, or the need to aim to continually strive to go longer and faster. I did not want to pit myself against anyone else. I found the rhythm of running soothing and allowed me to think things over and help gain perspective and direction, in the same way that dog walking also did for me later in life. Although others did try to goad me into competition and other distractions, I managed to keep things the way I liked it for life, just doing what I knew I could do without causing injury. Indeed, whenever I upped the mileage or speed for some reason, an injury was the inevitable result, and then I could not run at all which was frustrating and counterproductive. The fact that I am still running and enjoying it forty years later is testament to my approach, I always think.

I did train up and run the London Marathon twice just to see if I could manage the distance and I achieved times that I felt were acceptable, but I did not enjoy that type of running. The experiences of running the marathons in London were wonderful, with the vast crowds lining the streets providing atmosphere, encouragement, ambient music, and ribald comments. Even just little touches like those households who put up notices in their gardens imploring competitors not to use them as urinals were entertaining. Even on the second occasion, when training had not gone well so I was under-prepared, and I had a stomach upset on the day and so wasted half an hour on several toilet stops, it was enjoyable in a way. It was certainly a challenge that I felt glad I had got through, even if I did end up walking part of the distance. However, this last experience was the thing that set me against ever doing another one. Having a goal to reach by a particular time added a stress that detracted from my enjoyment of the run itself, and, besides, trying to train with a full-time job, out-of-hours commitments, a young family to attend to, and all the house and garden upkeep, was virtually impossible. I got no support from Rebekah, my first wife, who did not exercise at all and seemed unhappy with what I did. Much like work, she viewed my absence from the home on training runs to be time I should have been there with her. She never supported me when I was training for the marathons, and refused to attend either of them, or the Great North Run that I also ran. I found that the long runs and the training for them were an investment in time that I could not afford and having to perform on the day took away from the spontaneity that was part of the attraction. Just waking up and thinking that it seemed like a good day for a run was one of the simple pleasures that I take from life. My usual distances were three to five miles, and I could do the local annual ten kilometre run without too much problem, and I was happy with that. With my second wife Suzy, I found someone who shared this enjoyment, albeit she had to change her running environment from the cushioned treadmill in the gym that she was used to and move to the great outdoors with its varying surfaces. However, she found that she much preferred the outdoor running, and she would call out her welcome to all of the wildlife and domestic animals she passed as she ran. She, in her turn, slowly persuaded me into more appropriate running kit, away from the heavy cotton sweats and t-shirts that I habitually wore, and into lighter, more comfortable clothing that kept me warmer, and which wicked away the sweat, and so improved the experience for me. Heavy cotton, wet from rain or sweat, either sticking closely to me or swinging heavily with the motion of running, had never been a particularly pleasant part of the running experience. Even now I will still get a run in before work when I can, and cold weather running is more comfortable with the fleece-lined leggings I now have. I notice that a lot of guys wear a pair of shorts over theirs when they run, but I have never understood why. Perhaps they believe themselves to be so well-endowed that this is bound to be prominently shown in tight-fitting leg wear. If so, then they obvious have not run much in the cold. I find things retreat so much that I end up feeling that I have gained an extra pair of tonsils, and there is certainly nothing out there on show.

In running, as with so much else, I found that contentment with my lot was preferable to always striving for more. True, having the right equipment helped, but I always liked to get out in the fresh air and do some exercise. I enjoyed it even more when I had somebody close to share it with, and so I found Suzy to be, in this respect and so many others, an absolute godsend. We did not race each other. If we had to stop for some reason, then so be it. The commonest reason for this was to attend to some stricken wildlife, either to aid it or to remove its traumatised corpse from the lane as Suzy did not want it to be run over by anything else. I have several times been called by Suzy whilst she has been out running alone and come across something that needed attention, whether it be an injured rabbit or a dead deer. But most of the time we just jog along together. As time has passed and Suzy's distances have exceeded mine, we have changed so that she runs a circular route and I time running the same route in the opposite direction so that I meet her after she has completely roughly three quarters of the distance. That way I run half of what she does, and we are both happy.

CHAPTER 8

Unfortunately, my lack of experience with the other sex both before and during university had left me almost entirely clueless about women once I had left with my medical degree and gone out into the wider world. Of course, it is debatable hospitals count as the wider world as they were still something of an enclosed environment in which I spent most of my time and to which the outside world intruded in only certain ways. I had accommodation on site and was working long days with frequent evenings, nights and weekends on-call, and thus free time was limited and at a premium. The fact that I remained shy and uncomfortable socially did not help me in the least.

Having qualified with a 2:1 medical degree, I was not immediately a fully-fledged doctor but had to spend a year in what were then called pre-registration house jobs, in a role called a Junior Houseman. I had to spend six months on a surgical ward and the other six months in medicine, where the treatment was primarily medication rather than surgery or other interventions. These jobs were a requirement that had to be fulfilled in a suitable fashion and be duly signed off by the consultant that I had worked for, in order that I could then attain full registration with the General Medical Council and so go on to forge a career. A similar thing happens these days, but the grade of doctor is now called a Foundation Year Doctor and there are two years spent at this level. We did not benefit from the Working Time Directive and so long working hours were the norm, although I am aware that many hospitals put pressure on their doctors to waive their rights under the Directive when it came in and so still had to work a lot of hours, often unpaid for some of them. There are many memoirs available from other doctors about their experiences in such House Jobs, and mine were not significantly different to those of anybody else.

However, I did remember how tired I was, and how this must have impacted on my ability to do my job and make important decisions, especially when not supported by senior staff, and thus there was the potential for adverse impact upon my patients.

My first job was in surgery at a District General Hospital in East Anglia, and the six months were split into three months each with two different "firms," or teams of doctors led by a consultant. The first three months was in Urological Surgery where the consultant was public school educated and possessed a supreme confidence in his own ability which stopped just the right side of arrogance and so he engendered patients' confidence in him. The other three months was in a general and vascular surgical team with an equally talented surgeon but of a wholly different personality. He seemed a little socially awkward and, whilst a good boss to have, was unhappy in conversation outside that which was immediate clinical necessity. He was also a little uncomfortable around the nursing staff. The rumour was that he had once addressed a nursing sister as just "nurse" and she tore him off a strip for being disrespectful of her station on the ward where she was in charge. He clearly felt this keenly and thus addressed all nurses as "sister" in future for safety's sake, completely unaware that most of them felt he was being patronising by doing so. On one ward round a patient, who had been an inpatient for several weeks due to a series of complications to his surgery, broke down in tears whilst thanking the consultant for all he had done, and the consultant looked incredibly uncomfortable and did not know what to say. I saw this sort of surgeon so often I wondered whether that branch of medicine just attracted doctors who were happier dealing with patients who were asleep. I also recognised in that consultant something of my own social awkwardness and thus sympathised because, being the boss, he could not help being the centre of attention.

There were long, long days of routine ward work and there were frequent nights and weekends of being on-call, with working weeks of one hundred and twenty hours being a frequent occurrence. The nights and weekends were the worst as I was responsible for several wards of patients, and any new admissions to them, with just a senior house officer or registrar available to call upon if needed, whereas each of these wards had a whole team of doctors available to look after it during the day. Obviously there was the care of the acute admissions to deal with, but also complications arising from patients who had undergone routine surgery earlier in the day. Fate always seemed to dictate that these post-operative patients waited for their regular team of doctors to clock off before their condition suffered mammary elevation. i.e. they went tits up and needed some urgent intervention to prevent them going feet first. There was also the constant and unsettling sensation that one was flying by the seat of one's pants, with only limited confidence whilst experience grew, and having to react rapidly to changing situations and clinical priorities, and with constant demand. It was during these jobs that the National Health Service started to recoup some of the money that had been invested in me for my medical education. Not only were the hours long, but a standard working week was taken as being forty hours long, and I was paid the standard rate for that. The rest of the hours that I worked during the week were considered to be over-time, but rather than this attracting a higher rate of pay, I was instead paid at a rate of one-third of that I received for normal hours.

A weekend on-call for me in those early days meant me starting at eight o'clock on a Friday morning and having to be on-site and constantly available until six o'clock on the following Monday evening for several wards full of sick people. That is a straight eighty-two-hour shift with no designated breaks or guaranteed sleep. I know that junior doctors work long hard hours now but nothing like that. And I would be straight back onto the wards on the Tuesday morning as well – there were no days or half-days off to compensate. When on duty I would be taking calls from surrounding GP practices and the Accident and Emergency Department regarding admitting and dealing with the acute emergencies relevant to the department for which I was on-call. Another task for the duty doctor was that they had to carry the "crash" bleep, which meant I would be part of the small team who responded to emergency bleeps which went off when there was a cardiac arrest somewhere in the hospital. If the crash bleep sounded, I would be required to immediately drop anything that I was doing and run at top speed to the ward where the incident had happened, there to form part of the group of professionals attempting resuscitation on the hapless patient. There would be junior doctors, senior nurses, and anaesthetists on the team. A problem would occur if this bleep went off during a ward round as the presiding consultant would take a dim view of his most junior staff member (i.e., the one who was going to have to do all of the tasks that the consultant wanted done, and who would be making a note of them as we went) having to leave and run off, and several times refused permission for me to do so, leaving me then having to make excuses to the duty anaesthetist for my absence.

In my first job, during the run up to Christmas, I had to be on-call for five weekends out of six, as well as doing all of the usual week's duties and on-call commitments. The hospital that I worked in consisted of two blocks separated by a quarter-mile long corridor, which gradually sloped down and then up again along its length, and which was quite a run when I had to attend a crash call. Sod's Law always dictated that when the crash bleep sounded, I was working in the other block to the one in which the call originated, and so several long sprints a day left me even more tired than before. I would also become somewhat more malodorous with the running as well as constantly working in an environment kept warm for the comfort of the patients, especially as a duty weekend wore on. After all, one of the things you might be doing when the crash bleep sounded was taking a shower, and so these were rarely taken when on-call. It was easier to just wear surgical scrubs all the time and then change them when you noticed people starting to edge away in the lift. The more senior doctors on the team were theoretically available to help when the team was "on take" for acute admissions, but I quickly learnt that they considered that my job was to make sure that they were not disturbed out of hours if possible. After all, they seemed to reason, they had worked this apprenticeship themselves when younger and more junior, and so they wanted to reap the rewards now that this particular trial was over for them.

I had never been so tired. I felt that I had gained some experience but had not furthered my medical knowledge beyond understanding exactly what the job that I was employed to do consisted of, which was something that my medical school lectures had skilfully avoided. I did learn the practical application of some of what I had learnt at medical school, but there was certainly no element of formal teaching from the Consultants or Registrars during either of my junior placements, although that was meant to be a part of their role. I later enjoyed reading some of the books that came out by other former junior doctors about their experiences, and I marvelled at the incredulity of the public over what were, to me and my contemporaries, almost everyday events. I presume that nobody could genuinely appreciate what me and my battle-hardened colleagues had gone through, in the same way that I could not fully appreciate the experiences of other emergency workers. I did learn a lot about my own capabilities and resilience, as well as that of every other worker in the National Health Service, regardless of role or status, and I learnt even more about the resilience and fortitude in extremis of the general population.

One change that I have noticed through my career has been the drop in the number of nurses around. As a junior doctor on the wards, I was practically tripping over nurses at every turn. If I came onto a ward during morning report, there would be a flock of nurses seated around the nurses' station, like pigeons at a park bench, displaying different plumage according to their rank and experience, whilst the sister or nurse in charge would dispense titbits of information on each patient on the ward, such as how long they had been there, what sort of night they had passed, what would be happening to them today, etc. At the end of this report, they would rise as one to disperse to their allotted tasks. When I have visited wards more recently to visit somebody it has taken the keen eye of a dedicated twitcher to even spot a brief glimpse of a nurse as they flit rapidly from job to job as if they had a raptor on their tail, for they seem sadly depleted in number and under constant pressure of time.

It was during my first such junior job that I met the girl who was to later become my wife. I met her after the first couple of months, although apparently, I had been in her sights for a while by then. Rebekah had done her nurse training at the hospital where I was working and, having recently qualified as a Staff Nurse, she clearly felt that she was suitably placed to approach a doctor. She later related that her heart had gone out to me after she had to call me to her ward at six o'clock one Sunday morning during one of my weekends on call. It had been a busy Friday and Saturday and I was so tired by that time that I had fallen asleep at the front desk of the ward in the thirty seconds that it had taken her to fetch the paperwork for the patient she wanted me to see, my head cushioned on my arm. For my part, I was flattered to have been noticed and was willing to accompany her for a drink when she suggested it. We went to a pretty little riverside pub that she knew of, but whilst she was nicely dressed, I was just in a plaid shirt with rolled up sleeves, old jeans and the clumpy stockman's boots I had brought back with me from Australia. I got the feeling that she did not think that I had made much of an effort, but then I did not boast an extensive wardrobe, clothes and fashion having never really meant that much to me. We chatted well enough and found that we had a reasonable amount in common. It is not surprising considering that we were both in caring professions, but she liked jazz funk whilst I was still keen on rock music. However, this did not seem to be an insurmountable obstacle and so things went from there. Her parents lived up in Norfolk, and we went there to stay whenever we had a weekend off together. This seemed a bit of a trip at the time, but we would set off in my old Escort car after work on the Friday and return late on the Sunday evening, after a restful weekend and plenty of good food and jovial hospitality from Rebekah's parents. It was a chance for me to catch up on some sleep, but if it was felt that I had lain in long enough then the door would be opened and the household's Old English Sheepdog would be allowed in to say Good Morning, something that nobody could have managed to sleep through. Walking the dog around the quiet lanes nearby was also a good relaxing way to spend time.

The relationship survived a six-month separation whilst I undertook a job abroad, the second of my two junior jobs, and we subsequently settled in East Anglia where I started my training to become a General Practitioner, the direction that I had chosen for myself whilst at medical school and from which my hospital experiences had failed to divert me. I had also set my sights on East Anglia during my university days. One of the lads who had a room next to me in halls lived in the West Norfolk countryside, where his father was an estate manager. This friend was usually roped into a summer job by his father whereby he had to sell frozen vegetables from the farm from the back of a refrigerated truck at various spots around Norfolk. I had been invited to stay for a week and had accompanied him on his selling trips, helping him to load up the lorry and do some other lifting where needed. I then went off from every selling pitch to explore the local area, be that Norwich or several of the larger villages around, and we did some sightseeing together as he showed me around his home county. Whilst there I marvelled at the broad and open countryside, the variable coastline with cliffs, sand-dunes, shingle and vast beaches, and the huge expanse of sky. I did not want to go back to be near London again, and Norfolk seemed to be as good a place as any to put down some roots of my own.

The job that I took abroad was quite an experience of its own. It was in the civilian hospital in Gibraltar, St Bernard's, and at the time, it felt almost third world in its setup and equipment. The hospital was situated a reasonable distance up the hill from the main street and was reached by a steep ramp-like road. The

Accident and Emergency department was on the left and up some stairs and linked to the main hospital by a covered corridor above the road access. The rest of the hospital was arranged in a square, with a small footprint but several stories high. The corridor from the A&E met the middle of one side of the square, and there was a taller block directly opposite. This taller block held most of the wards, including the two Geriatric wards in the lower levels into which I delved regularly to undertake ward-rounds although I was rarely accompanied there by the consultants. The patients on these wards seemed to change very little, and so they seemed to function as nursing homes more than hospital wards. The blocks on each side of the square were a few storeys lower than this ward block, and in the far-right corner was angled an accommodation block that linked to the rest. There were three junior doctors in all, me in medicine and two others in the surgical department. There was also one Senior House Officer, the grade one reached having completed the year of probation and been fully registered with the General Medical Council. He worked in the Accident and Emergency department where his experience of all aspects of medicine would be best used. All these doctors were from the UK, two from the same part of Scotland, whilst me and the Senior Houseman were from England. There were three consultants that we worked for and who were resident on the Rock, two physicians and one general surgeon. To complement these staff, there were visiting surgeons who were based at the military hospital at the tip of Gibraltar, who performed Obstetrics and Gynaecology, and Orthopaedics respectively. Apart from specialist consultants, such as for Ear, Nose and Throat, and Neurology, who visited from the UK a few times a year, this was the hospital medical team for the entire population, although there was also a private practice that patients could attend. Anyone who was seriously ill, especially if they needed any kind of complex procedure or intensive care, essentially had to be evacuated to the UK by air for that treatment. Although there was a Cardiac Ward, this just meant that somebody was keeping a better eye on them than on the general ward, and it bore no more likeness to a UK Coronary Care Unit than the general wards did. Admission to this ward meant that there was an ECG monitor for each person and someone in constant attention who noticed if they sounded and summoned help. There were none of the interventions that one would otherwise expect on such a unit in the UK, such as pacemakers, stents and coronary angiography, and I felt that the mortality rate generally seemed un-necessarily high. The medical care for service personnel was entirely separate to that for the population.

I did subsequently revisit Gibraltar some thirty years later but did not go back to the hospital for a look. However, I am aware that a big new hospital has been built down by the marina and harbour now, with most of the windows looking out towards the sea, albeit no longer from on high but sitting just above a rocky shoreline. The main town still jostled right up to the foot of the green and dramatic rise of the Rock itself, but it had changed. The former hostel for Moroccan workers at the harbour end of the main street had been changed to a development of artisan shops, and the main street itself had been pedestrianised instead of having two lanes of bad-tempered traffic to negotiate. Also, the new hospital was part of a large new development encircling the port.

Gibraltar itself I had enjoyed a lot. I was not really sure why I had applied for the job in the first place, but I thought it was probably a reluctance to let go of the sense of independence that I had found when I went to Australia. I had a colleague in my year at medical school who had family in Gibraltar, and who was going out to do the job for the six months before I went, and I had heard about the vacancy from him. It sounded exciting and new, and I was not at all sure when, if ever, I would have the chance to do anything similar again. I had chosen my career in General Practice by this time, and so the job would not go against me, indeed, it would show some element of the sort of skills and autonomy that General Practice required. Had I wanted to become a career physician or surgeon, such a job would have been career suicide as it would not have been up to the sort of standard that eminent consultants would want to see from their upcoming juniors. As time would tell, I never did have the opportunity to do anything remotely like that again, and so never looked back on my time there with regret, just a sense of being thankful that I had survived it and having gained some valuable experience there.

The hospital always looked somewhat hemmed in by the buildings that surrounded it, as did everywhere in the town. All the junior staff had accommodation in the block on one corner of the hospital, and when I looked out of the side window I felt as if I could pick a flower from the window box of the property just across the street. However, if I looked in another direction the slope just fell away, and I had a wonderful view of the harbour and the sea. This was even better from the roof of the building, where there was a little room that served as a laundry, and clothes could be hung from lines in the sun, hopefully upwind from the smuts from the hospital boiler chimney that opened onto the same roof. Although we were clearly intended to use the roof for this purpose, there was no precaution such as barriers or handrails up there and one could walk right to the edge of the flat roof and look down four or five stories into the central quadrangle. The crossing between the accommodation block and the main ward block was just a plank laid from one flat roof to another. Fortunately, the distance was short, and it only needed a step or two before you were across.

Exploration showed that all the roads in Gibraltar town seemed narrow and twisty. Cars were variously parked or abandoned along the sides and corners of every thoroughfare, making any passage or negotiation tricky, especially as this was many years before the advent of parking sensors in cars. The ambulance, just the one, was a small van with no medical equipment on board, just a stretcher and drivers with a fierce determination to get the stricken patient to the hospital as quickly as possible. This was not made easy because nobody seemed to take any notice of the fact that the siren was blaring loudly and certainly did not seem to be in any hurry to get out of the ambulance's way. Many of the buildings along busy streets, and most of the corners everywhere, bore the scars of traffic passing too close, and most of the vehicles in the town looked battered and past their best.

I was happy to live there for a while but would not have liked to be there permanently, as all aspects of life there seemed to go against my "play by the rules" mentality, and the general mañana attitude was frustrating and exhausting. When I was there, the border with Spain had been newly opened after a prolonged closure of many years due to tensions between the UK and Spain over sovereignty of the colony, a disagreement that continues to this day. I felt that there was some duplicity in the Spanish position, as they were unhappy at having a British enclave in what they considered to be Spain, whilst they themselves had Ceuta in North Africa, directly across the Strait, which worked in entirely the same way, but with Spain in charge of a promontory and city on the edge of a different continent.

Nevertheless, the border was open, and I would walk across to La Linea, the town across the border in the Spanish province of Andalucía, to get fresh produce from the market, and for evenings out. One of my favourites was to go to a small place that did calzone pizza, or plates piled high with bread-crumbed fried prawns, with a liberal dusting of salt, accompanied by cold beer or three. I certainly preferred that ambience to the pubs full of squaddies back on the Rock, however much they might have been reminders of home. Indeed, I was not sure that reminders of home were what I needed. That was not the point of getting away in the first place, and things were never the same as they would have been at home anyway. The miniscule Marks and Spencer store in the main street just seemed incongruous rather than reassuring. The Marina area had received a face-lift before I arrived and I liked that environment, but mostly because it was continental in feel rather than British. The Governor's Residence and change of guard outside was popular with tourists but, again, was that really necessary? Most locals that I spoke to were proud to be British and did not need such demonstrations to support that notion. The flag was sufficient for them, and possibly the language. However, that was a problem in itself. I knew some Spanish, but it did not help me with the local dialect nor the Spanglish way that Gibraltarians had of conversing, in which the two languages were mixed within the same sentence. It was as if the speaker had arranged two piles of cards, one where each card contained a word necessary for the conversation in English, and a similar one in Spanish, and then shuffled them and spoke the sentence formed when they were dealt out a hand from that resulting pack. During ward rounds, having a member of the nursing staff present was always vital to act as interpreter. There was also short-hand Spanish used. I used to hear a question asked of every patient, that sounded like "Tommy whore?" When asked of a female patient it sounded like she was being accused of extra-curricular services to members of the garrison. It had to be explained that the question was actually a slang version of "Est tu mejor?" which essentially meant "Are you feeling better?"

The walk to the border was bizarre in that the runway for the airport crossed the road leading between border with Spain and the main street of the town. This meant that both pedestrians and traffic were held up for some time whilst an aircraft took off or landed, which I somehow found a quaint and charming arrangement. I started the job in February, when it was rather cold despite being on the Mediterranean coast, and I found that I could really have done with some warmer clothing. However, as Spring subsequently came and then gave way to Summer, the weather got hotter and hotter as the days lengthened. There were only a few beaches on Gibraltar, most of the coast being rocky and inaccessible. Because of this, such beaches as there were became crammed on sunny days, but they were usually only in the sun for part of the day because of the enormous shadow that Gibraltar itself cast upon the ground around it as the sun progressed from East to West across the sky, making the Rock like some giant sundial. This caused large parts of the population to move around the coast through the days looking for a sunny spot, whilst the watermark of humanity slowly moved across the beach ahead of the advancing shade, until all finally deserted it for a sunnier spot or some refreshment.

Then there were the days of Levanter, when a cloud formed around the upper slopes of the Rock, like a mink wrap around the shoulders of a distinguished and formidable lady, but with the effect of blocking out sunshine for all but the furthest tip of the land, known as Europa Point, and which was part of the military area. On those days, if unable to leave to seek the sunshine, one just had to sit under the oppressive cloak of that cloud and watch the sun-drenched coast of Spain just across the bay. It was amazing just how many otherwise glorious days were lost under that covering, which was formed by a particular set of sea and wind conditions but was nonetheless frustrating for all of that. I also felt that this suffocation by the cloud was like the way I had felt when depressed at university, feeling as if I were smothered and unable to free myself from the feeling, whilst I could see others enjoying themselves not too far away, but out of reach. Fortunately, the depression itself did not return, and never has, although the Levanter kept turning up like a bad penny on my days off throughout my time there.

Rebekah came out to visit Gibraltar whilst I was there, the first time being a matter of weeks after I had arrived, and she announced herself to be dissatisfied. She said that she had expected me to have discovered all the hidden gems of restaurants and bars to take her to whilst she was there. I tried to explain that actually I was working extremely hard, as were we all, as there were only four junior staff for the whole hospital. We had barely had any social life at all since our own arrival and I would have liked nothing better than to have had time to discover all these quaint places to eat and drink at my own leisure. She was appeased by the purchase of some leather clothing from the markets in Tangiers, but subsequently stated that did not want to return there because she felt it looked filthy and was full of children who pulled at her clothing and wanted hand-outs. She also did not want to see another haunch of animal hung up in the heat and flies with the animal's testicle still dangling from it. Neither did she want to eat anything there for fear of picking up something unpleasant, despite a meal from a reputable outlet being built into the cost of the day trip that we had taken. However, I was not too displeased with this idea of not going back as the trip we had taken across the Strait from Gibraltar to Morocco by motor catamaran ferry had been bumpy and nauseating despite the sea appearing reasonably calm. The idea that we might hit a day with more of a swell did not bear thinking about, and the atmosphere was not helped by there being many Moroccan workers huddled up on the seats in misery at their own seasickness or giving vent to their nausea over the rear gunwale amongst the diesel exhaust from the engines.

For Rebekah's second visit to Gibraltar, I took some time out and did something different and a little more adventurous. I hired a car which we picked up across the border, and I drove us both across Andalucía towards Portugal, where we boarded a ferry to take us across the Guadiana River which forms the border between the two countries at that point. We then motored along the Algarve to the charming town of Albufeira. At least, it was charming then. The whole area, including this town, was much less busy and built up then than it is now. We parked in the town and went to the Tourist Information centre whose staff directed us to a guest house with a vacancy and so we arranged to stay there for the week. We had a wonderful time, with sunbathing all day, a pool on the roof of the guest house for dips to make a change from the beach, and a restaurant downstairs which served the freshest of seafood. The spontaneity of the trip made it all the better, and I often looked back at it as one of the best times that we ever shared together. It was a shame that things never seemed as good between us again, but life was free and uncomplicated at that point, and that had much to do with it. The eventual return to the UK and need to pursue a career subsequently added stresses and strains that I applied myself to but did not often manage to look up from them to see where exactly I was going. Perhaps I had allowed Rebekah to steer too much, and this turned out to be in a direction that I was not so keen to go in. The decisions we made always seemed to be a compromise on my intended direction, somehow, and I never felt that I was captain of my own ship.

The Rock itself had various things to explore. The Apes (which are really macaque monkeys from Africa) had the same nonchalant vandalism that I had previously seen amongst the inmates of safari parks in the UK, with them eating, defaecating, fornicating, and wilfully destroying with equal vigour and candour. Tourists regularly turned up in the hospital's small Accident and Emergency Department with bites to show where they had tried to boss the monkeys and come off worse. Then there were the Mediterranean Steps to explore. Starting some half-way up the twisting roads to the summit, they formed a trail of rough path and steep steps which were cut into the mount and led around to the more sheer side of the rock, where the water capture surfaces were. This was an energetic trek up towards the summit, with spectacular views on the way, and the return trip to the bottom was by way of the twisting roads again. There were also siege tunnels, fortifications, including old ones dating from Moorish times, and underground caverns to explore. This could be done with ropes and much scrabbling, which was quite an adventure with narrow ledges to be walked along next to utterly still water of seemingly infinite depth, but the largest cavern was a venue for music concerts by military bands. One of the favourite haunts on the Rock of me and my contemporaries was an eatery that seemed tiny from the outside, but whose inside had literally been excavated into rock behind, forming a den that was cosy and atmospheric, serving food that could scarcely be contained by the plates that bore it, whether it be a steak or a Dover sole, which choice seemed to encompass the whole menu.

CHAPTER 9

Training to be a General Practitioner took several years of work and consisted of several different six-month posts as a Senior House Officer in various medical specialities, as well as two six-month stints as a General Practitioner Registrar in practice with an experienced partner supervising. As with much of the country, there was a local Vocational Training Scheme in Norfolk. This was where a ready-made rotation of suitable jobs was organised for the candidates by the local deanery so that the doctor knew exactly what jobs they were going to do, and when, over a three-year period. The set-up also meant that, when the doctors were in their training practices, they were given a half-day a week out of the practice to attend a series of lectures and demonstrations at the further education centre of the local hospital. There was great demand and competition for places on the scheme and for General Practice jobs in those days, and I failed to gain one when I applied and underwent interview. Undaunted I decided that I would put my own scheme together by applying for appropriate hospital jobs and General Practice training places on an individual basis and off my own back. Training places would have to be approved by the local deanery anyway so there should have been no risk of a substandard attachment. However, putting together my own scheme meant that I was technically going to be unemployed every six months and would need to start applying for my next job before I was even half-way through the current one, which made for a patchy-looking job history. This fact caused problems with getting a mortgage at first, but they were more enlightened and enabling times for banks and so patient explanation of both the process and the potential future job security meant that a mortgage was ultimately secured to allow myself and Rebekah to buy our first home together. This was a two-bedroomed bungalow that had been built in the 1970s in a village on the river Bure at the edge of the complex of the Norfolk Broads, just down the road from where I had secured my first job as a trainee GP. Although the riverside village in which we lived was lovely at any time of year, it became so full of visitors in the summer that we could never really enjoy it. The river Bure was just a short walk away down the hill from our bungalow, with a lovely open grassy bank area and two pubs which nestled cheek by jowl on the riverbank. It was a wonderful place to relax in the sunshine, but was considered such by so many people, both from near and afar, that it became very crowded and so rather lost its charm on such days. Like so many people who live in areas of tourist potential, we found ourselves unable to enjoy the benefits on our doorstep but had, instead, to travel to less well-known spots in the area for our own leisure.

As mentioned, my first training job in General Practice was similarly on the Broads but further along the river, in a town whose population swelled immensely from Spring to Autumn as holidaymakers rushed to stay in cabins along the riverfronts and hire boats to cruise the waterways for anything from a few hours to a few weeks at a time. The town, which was really two towns twinned across the river Bure, had a commerce that seemed to be dominated by just one man, as his name was emblazoned across the top of nearly every shop along the High Street at the time. It was my first experience of General Practice, and I was well looked after in terms of a gradual introduction to patient consultations, leading eventually to doing my own clinics and some of the on-call commitment of the practice. This meant that I was the doctor who was called when the Surgery was shut in the evenings, overnight, and at weekends, and would have to be available to assist in any medical problem that arose. I was supported on these occasions by one of the partners who would be available on the end of a phone, although this would have to be a landline as there were no mobile phones in those days. If I were attending a patient who did not own a phone, then I might have to knock on a neighbour's door or look for a call box to ring from. If the partner was not immediately available, then I would have to leave a message and then hang around either place waiting for a call back.

There were four partners, and the group was long-established, so they knew each other's personalities and foibles well enough and got along well as a team. They had hugely different personalities but, whilst they all had their own characters, what united them, in my eyes, was apparent wealth. They had large rambling houses, sent children to public school, had frequent holidays abroad, and generally lived what appeared to be wonderfully comfortable lives. I hoped that this would bode well for my own prospects. What I did not know at the time, was that this was all destined to change quite quickly, so that, by the time I reached the age that they had been at the time, neither I nor any of my contemporaries could aspire to anything like that income or lifestyle.

In this Broads medical practice there was a central Surgery where most of the work was done, and which was the nerve centre of medical and administrative tasks. However, there were also four outlying morning surgeries held each week, one by each of the partners, and I took a turn with each of these. These were held in villages towards the periphery of the Practice area, and utilised various buildings or rooms in community centres where the patients could be seen. However, because these facilities were not set up for this purpose, equipment was extremely basic as it had to fit into the doctor's bag, and so only simple problems could be dealt with. Similarly, only simple procedures could be done, such as administering influenza vaccinations. Anything requiring equipment or testing needed to be referred to the central surgery for follow-up. Indeed, even physical examinations could be perfunctory as the lack of heating in the buildings did little to encourage the patients to disrobe appropriately. I got used to having my request to examine somebody's chest being met with the patient undoing a single button on their shirt or blouse and pulling the two sides apart to reveal a kite-shaped patch of skin overlying the breastbone supposedly to allow my thorough assessment of their respiratory system. My requests for better access to their chest wall were met with comments along the lines that their usual, *more experienced*, doctor managed perfectly well with just that, so why could I not? Despite the significant shortcomings of these outlying clinics, the patients all loved them and each venue, and thus each partner, had a regular clientele of its own. I have to admit the standard of medicine was not all it could have been in these places, as there were no facilities for proper examination of patients, and areas of the body seemed to be examined through layers of clothing that would surely muffle any extra sound being listened for or any sign palpated for, but I held my tongue. This was all part of the learning experience, and I did not have to follow suit in my own future if I did not wish to. I felt that the education experience in GP training was probably not intended to be two-way and telling somebody more senior that they had been doing something wrong for a couple of decades never goes down too well.

There were other things within that first practice that belonged to an earlier time too and would certainly not happen today. One of these was the Wednesday lunch. The surgery had its own dispensary from which it could dispense prescribed drugs to any of its patients who lived more than a mile from a pharmacy, which was most of them given its rural setting. The dispensary could buy in medicines and then reclaim the cost of those that it dispensed from the local health authority according to a defined tariff list published centrally. If the drugs cost less than the reimbursed tariff then they kept the profit, so deals with drug companies upon the price of their drugs were worth having and contributed significantly to the individual doctor's incomes. Therefore, they had remarkably close links with a variety of drug company representatives who wished to do business with the team and have their own medications stocked and prescribed by them. Part of this arrangement was that the partners would be taken out for a three-course lunch at a local hotel each Wednesday by one representative or another, which took a large chunk of time out of the working day, and which was followed by a truncated afternoon surgery. This was performed by the duty doctor for that day alone, whilst the others finished the day early. I was invited along to these events too, even though I would not be able to influence the purchasing of medications at the surgery. I believed that the reps had an eye on me for business in the future. Of course, such things are not possible now and currently I have not had so much as a pen or post-it note from a drug rep for some years, but at the time I remembered my father and the Christmas hampers and did not feel that such things were all that strange. Rewards for patronage seemed to be the way that business was done in all spheres of life. The six-month stint I did there passed quickly, and I felt that I had learned a lot from the experience, especially about how medicine in General Practice differed from that in hospitals, which had been my only experience up until that point.

The hospital jobs that I chose to do as part of my training covered the full gamut of experience that would be relevant to General Practice. These jobs were therefore in Medicine for the Elderly, where I spent a year, Obstetrics and Gynaecology, another year, and six months each in Paediatrics, Psychiatry (where, I had to be honest, it was often difficult to tell the patients from the staff at a glance, as they dressed to be similar to, rather than stand out from those in their care), Rheumatology, and Ear, Nose and Throat. These last two jobs were not to be found on most structured vocational training rotations, but I felt them to be important, and experience showed them to have been invaluable as these areas of medicine accounted for a significant percentage of my workload as a GP.

The Medicine for the Elderly jobs were also good training, as they encompassed elements of social care and provision that were part of my everyday vocabulary as a GP. I knew roughly what I was in for on the first day when I arrived on the ward, only to be immediately ushered behind a curtain by the nurse in charge for the first job of the day which was to confirm the death of one of the patients who had passed away overnight. It could not have been a less auspicious start, but was certainly representative of my time there, as winter wore on and took its grim harvest from the crop of frail elderly folk of Norfolk. In medical school I had learned a lot about the pathophysiology of different medical conditions, from hypertension to angina, heart failure to emphysema, diabetes to dementia, but from the patients on these wards I learned what it was like to live with these conditions and to manage them, from the perspective of patient, carer and doctor. Similarly, I found that the medical perspective to every condition was that there had to be some intervention that would treat it, whereas many patients exhibited the more phlegmatic opinion that this was who they were now, and they must make the best of the hand that life had dealt them. To see so many patients bear considerable discomfort and disability with such dignity was very humbling, especially as it was usually accompanied by an acceptance of their lot and the strong desire to just "Keep on a-doin' young man" as they would frequently say in their local dialect. It was also concerning that some of them were exposed to medical interventions that were either unhelpful or even harming, just so that the medical fraternity could reassure themselves that they had done everything that they could. Skilled and watchful inactivity was not part of hospital medicine, it seemed. It was another exceptionally good grounding for a Primary Care career where the long-term management and monitoring of a patient's health and illness were the very foundations of practice.

It was during this job that I received probably the best compliment that I have ever had, but also the most concerning. I had been called in the night to an elderly lady who had developed crushing heart failure, where the heart muscle essentially decides that it has had enough of the whole regular pumping thing and downs tools to the extent that its beats are weak and ineffectual, leading to back-pressure which causes acute accumulation of fluid in the lungs, dramatically affecting oxygen absorption and causing extreme distress. I battled with this using oxygen and intravenous medication for an hour or so, but she was not responding, and her condition deteriorated. She was not for resuscitation and so, when I realised that we were approaching the end of the road, I downed tools myself, sat on the edge of her bed, and held her hand. She gripped it with significantly more muscular effort than her myocardium had exhibited and was clearly terrified. I spoke to her in what I hoped was a gentle and reassuring tone, and continued my firm grip of her hand, and watched as she lost her unequal struggle to hold on to life. I waited a few minutes more, still holding her hand, and then went through the procedure to confirm life extinct and pronounce her death. The ward Sister later told me that a nurse who was in attendance had been impressed by my compassion, although I felt that I had merely done the minimum that would be considered reasonable. The cause for my concern is that, if that was considered so noteworthy, then just what had she seen other doctors do in similar circumstances.

Looking back, I can see that there was no consideration of neurodiversity in the elderly population, though it must surely have existed. Discharge plans for patients would include arrangements for them to attend day-care centres and lunch clubs with no consideration of whether this what they wanted. If they declined to go then there was no alternative. I know that I would not want to attend such places, crammed onto minibuses to get there and back, but I would, on the other hand, love to have access to audio books or a mobile library on a regular basis instead. These were not options that ever came up in strategy meetings and I am not sure that they do even to this day. So much for patient-centred care.

One other aspect that I developed during this time was a sense of spirituality. Raised as Church of England, though my mother's background was that of Scottish Presbyterian, I could not say that I was in any way religious, and I admitted to no such affiliation. However, my job meant that I was present at the moment of death of several patients, and I considered this to be the ultimate privilege of my position. I noticed that, on these occasions, there was identifiably a moment which I referred to as "Elvis has left the building," whereby some inner presence was recognisable in a body at one moment, even in an unconscious or insensible patient, but was obviously gone the next. I was certain that the human body was essentially a home for this presence, however one might refer to it, but that the two were intimately connected during life. However, at the moment of death, this "essence of self" appeared to leave the body it had inhabited, to what destination I had no idea, and to what end, I similarly did not know. However, I could readily understand man's need to construct some way of explaining this phenomenon.

Later in my career, whilst working as a university lecturer, I was charged with trying to explain this phenomenon of self and spirituality to undergraduates who had to learn about its relevance to managing patients as they approached the end of their lives. One of the ways I did this was to show a You Tube video of part of an episode of the sitcom Only Fool's and Horses. In this, the character of Trigger, a road sweeper, was explaining how he had been awarded a medal for keeping the same broom for twenty years, and then pointed out that it had had seventeen new heads and fourteen new handles in that time. It was then asked of him how it could be the same broom at which he held up they newspaper bearing his photo and said that here was a picture of it so what more evidence did they need? I would then point out to the students that their bodies and the metabolic processes within were not static but were essentially unstable systems that required constant energy and nutrients for upkeep and that elements of all parts of their bodies and organs would be replaced many times over during their lifetime. Despite this, like the entity that was Trigger's broom in the photo, there remained, throughout these changes and renewals, an individual that they identified as themself. I asked them to consider what they thought this might consist of if the apparatus that carried it changed so much, or whether the two were actually the same thing. What was the relationship between the two, were they inherently linked, were they mutually dependent or could one exist without the other and, if so, then where? I also related the large number of elderly patients who report that, inside, they still feel twenty-one, it is just their ageing body that lets them down. So, did the students identify with that from their own experience and how did it make them feel about the relationship between the inner self and the body? Though I could offer no definitive answers to any of these questions, they stimulated much discussion and thought, which was the whole point of the exercise.

Towards the end of his life, my father related several episodes that had occurred when he had felt himself floating up from where he sat and found that he was looking down at himself still seated in his chair. Far from experiencing any enlightenment or sense of peace during these, he declared himself to be petrified and desperate to return to his corporeal body. Neither he nor I knew what to make of these, and I suspect that anybody reading about them will interpret them in the light of what they already believe, be it the presence of a soul and an afterlife or episodes of cerebral hypoxia. We call that cognitive bias in the trade. I guess we will all find out the truth eventually.

At the time of my General Practice training in the 1980s, the practice of mothers delivering their babies at home was still reasonably common, and so obstetric experience was an absolute requirement. I enjoyed my time in the department of Obstetrics and Gynaecology, although the former element was scary and demanding at times. I found the antenatal clinic to be the most uplifting and joyful clinic I had ever attended, notwithstanding the occasional tragedies that occurred in some pregnancies. The whole ethos within such clinics was a positive one for a welcome and happy situation, with something to look forward to at the end. Also, rather than there being a medical condition that had to be treated, this was a time-limited condition that merely had to be observed, or occasionally managed, to optimise the outcome for both mother and baby. This was so different from the pervasive sense of worry and despair that accompanied most significant and long-term medical conditions that required patients to attend other outpatient clinics at the hospitals. The other thing that was very different was the experience of the actual deliveries at the end of pregnancy. Uncomplicated deliveries in experienced mothers were all managed by the midwives alone, and the most complicated ones by the senior doctors on the team, although I was frequently called in to help in theatre with Caesarean section deliveries, often at short notice and in something of a rush. The deliveries that I was most involved with were the simple forceps deliveries, where mother had become exhausted with the process of pushing, or the stress of the birth was adversely affecting baby and this was being shown in the baby's heart rate, and baby just needed a little lift out to help deliver them into the world. I usually felt myself to be an unwelcome outsider at these births, for all that I was there to help bring it to a satisfactory conclusion. Usually, the mother and midwife had developed their relationship over several hours of labour with the hope of a normal birth to come, and my arrival signalled the failure of this and the imposition of a different approach. This new approach was also much more demonstratively intrusive, commanding, and medical, with stirrups for the woman's feet, and gowns and gloves for me, rendering me an almost sinister but certainly anonymous presence. The procedure was carried out with the patient in the so-called lithotomy position, so named after the Greek *lithso*, meaning stone, and *tomos*, meaning to cut. This was because this had been the position favoured for the removal of bladder stones, a once common affliction, via an incision made into the perineum and then on into the bladder. It required the lady to be lying on her back and to have her legs supported in an open position with hips and knees bent which was attained by placing her feet in hooped stirrups which were attached to metal posts that slotted into holes positioned at each side of the bed. Then the lower quarter of the hospital bed could be removed so that I could sit or stand there instead, leaving the expectant mother cruelly exposed and feeling as if she were lying up against the edge of a precipice. It was no surprise to me that, for the rest of my career when tentatively suggesting the need for a potentially embarrassing intimate examination to a female patient, a common reply was that they had given birth and were therefore left with no shred of dignity remaining, and that they were also incapable of embarrassment in front of a medical professional of any sort.

For the forceps procedure, and unless the patient had an epidural anaesthetic in place, I had to administer a pudendal block, which is the injection of local anaesthetic around the pudendal nerve in the pelvis, to numb the area before I could do anything towards helping to get baby out into the world. The local anaesthetic would be drawn up into a syringe, and a long needle was attached to the end with a metal guard over it that had a metal ring halfway along it. The idea was that I had to align my index finger along the needle and through this ring whilst holding the syringe. I then had to introduce the finger and needle between the crowning head of baby and the mother's pelvic wall until I could locate the ischial spine on the posterior aspect of the body of the pelvic bone, as this is where the pudendal nerve reliably runs. Once there, I could advance the needle from its covering and under the surface tissues to infiltrate some local anaesthetic around the nerve to block its transmission of sensory and pain signals and thus reliably numb the perineal area. This had to be done on both sides of the pelvis to numb the whole genital area, and I frequently found myself having to stand between the open legs of a lady I had only just met, wearing a hat, mask, gloves, and gown, trying to make small talk whilst I waited several minutes for the local anaesthetic to take effect, whilst she continued to have intermittent painful uterine contractions. Only when the numbness had spread to a satisfactory extent could I then slip the spoon-like forceps into place, one on each side of the baby's head, and bring the handles together to interlock so that I could hold them both together and apply traction to the baby in time with the next uterine contraction to advance the delivery. Then, just as the baby's head was making sudden and rapid progress towards the outside world, I would need apply some counter-pressure to the head for a second and then perform an episiotomy, a cut to the mother's perineum, which widened the way out of the birth canal and prevented the risk of that area tearing uncontrollably due to the width of the baby's head enveloped in the metallic crown it now wore. If this cut were not made, thus controlling what damage was done to the perineal area, it could tear in an unpredictable and uncontrolled way and cause damage to the muscles that close off the rectum, leaving the mother with the long-term risk of faecal incontinence. I would also have to check that the umbilical cord was not wrapped around baby's neck before attempting to deliver it.

Once baby had been safely delivered onto the mother's tummy and the forceps removed and placed back onto the shiny surgical trolley from whence they had come, I could go about clamping and cutting the cord, or waiting until the pulsation in its all-too-visible vessels had subsided before cutting. This would release the baby from its tether to the mother's womb and allow her to have her first proper physical contact with it. Then, when the uterus started to contract strongly again, usually under the influence of an intramuscular injection given for that purpose, it sheared the placenta from its anchorage to the inside wall of the uterus and I could then deliver that too by gentle traction on the cut end of the umbilical cord whilst applying gentle counter pressure to the body of the uterus by pressing on the lower anterior abdominal wall. That was all very satisfying, and the part of my intervention where I really felt that I had made a difference, but it was followed by my least favourite part for I then had to stitch up that episiotomy cut that I had made.

I would find myself sitting on a tiny stool between the mother's ever-open legs, trying to accurately suture back together that which I had put asunder, ever mindful of the need to do a decent job for the future comfort as well as continued enjoyable marital relations for the lady concerned. I had helped the surgeons in the Gynaecology operating theatres with subsequent late repairs when this suturing had been badly done in the past and I did not want to make a hash of it, regardless of whether this was the sixth time I had done it that shift and it was now in the small hours of the morning, and I had not eaten or drunk anything for hours, let alone had any sleep. By the time I was engaged in this part of the process the mother's endorphin rush from the delivery had passed, her legs and back were cramping and aching from the length of time she had been in the stirrups, she wanted to enjoy the baby, the local anaesthetic had begun to wear off and needed topping up, and nobody really wanted me there any longer. To say that it taxed my small talk to keep going through this exacting task without just grunting replies is to seriously understate the task I faced. Also, I often perceived waves of naked hostility coming from the male partners of the new mothers, who were clearly wondering why that bloke in the mask had to spend *quite* so much time with his nose up close to his partner's fanny. In fact, I felt about as welcome as a fart in a lift. But I got it done, and I was to find that most medical situations, whether good or bad, had this other side that only became apparent once you did the job. Whilst every good situation had an unwelcome element which could appear from nowhere, so a spark of humanity or humour could be found in the darkest of hours. Having gone through all of that, I only ended up delivering half a dozen babies for mothers at their homes once I was a GP, by which time the trend was diminishing, and community midwives were doing the vast majority anyway. In similar ways, the march of progress often seemed to outstrip the preparations made for my future practice, with hard worn experience becoming obsolete whilst there were always new methods and protocols to be learned. However, Rebekah was pregnant with Rose by this point in my career and so she was, at least, assured of the best care from the department in which her husband worked.

Maternity care in General Practice has also changed throughout my career. When I first started, a lady would come to the surgery to have her pregnancy confirmed, at which point she would arrange a booking appointment with me. This took half an hour and included paperwork to be filled, explanations to be given, blood to be taken, and literature and reference points dispensed. I would then see her every month until thirty weeks had passed, during which time she would also have been to the antenatal clinic and had contact with her midwife. After thirty weeks I would see her every two weeks until the thirty-eighth week, and then weekly until delivery occurred, and then see her afterwards. Nowadays pregnancy is confirmed by home testing and midwives deal with everything else. I will not see her until she brings her offspring to me for a post-natal check at six to eight weeks of age. I cannot help feeling that something important has been lost for both parties in these changes.

The other half of this job was in Gynaecology, which encompassed all problems relating to female anatomy and reproductive organs, and any pregnancy of less than 24 weeks in duration. Much of my time was spent dealing with urgent cases of abdominal or pelvic pain, with or without vaginal bleeding, from medical causes or threatened miscarriages. I had to admit these patients, assess them by taking a history and doing any examination or investigations that were needed, and make a diagnosis. A sizeable number of them required a procedure to remove retained material from the uterus, called a dilatation and curettage. I would then have to organise theatre time for the procedure and an anaesthetist to apply the general anaesthetic needed. Often calls would come in so fast that I was so busy going from one patient to another that I did not have time to arrange the theatre until later in the day by which time a small list had accumulated, at which the duty anaesthetist would often be a bit sniffy about me "saving up" all of my emergencies to do in one go. I would have to undertake these procedures myself, all whilst still having to be available for incoming calls from GPs and A&E.

The next job that I took was in Ear, Nose and Throat Surgery, known as ENT, to most, and as Otorhinolaryngology to the cognoscenti. I had realised that I had little grounding in this speciality previously but that it formed a large part of GP work. Whilst I was in the clinical years at medical school, there were certain "Cinderella" subjects that barely got any coverage in the curriculum and ENT was one such. It fell into a group of medical specialities referred to as Specials, which comprised ENT, ophthalmology, rheumatology, and dermatology. As students, we only had two weeks of exposure to these four broad and quite different disciplines in all of the five years that we spent in medical training. This two-week period fell in our final year and was partially sacrificed to allow more revision of the key areas in preparation for the final exams that fell in the same year. Those students who were intent on careers in General Medicine or General Surgery may not have mourned this lost opportunity, for there would be much less need for experience in them within these broad disciplines. However, for those students whose career paths led in the direction of General Practice, where these four disciplines could be guaranteed to form a significant part of every-day consultations, it was a noticeable and regrettable deficiency in our training. I had done my first General Practice training job by this time, and I was not full of confidence that even my trainer there had known his own way around an ear, nose, and throat examination. I did not feel that I had learnt much beyond the strategy of throwing antibiotics or steroids, or both, in the general direction of any problem within those areas, either as tablets, drops or sprays, and so I felt I needed to be better equipped in both knowledge and skills.

The job in ENT was in the same hospital as the Obstetrics and Gynaecology job, an institution now long since razed to make way for city centre housing, and replaced by a newer, but considerably smaller, hospital on the outskirts of Norwich. My role was Senior House officer but, as there were no Junior House Officers in this discipline, I remained on the lowest rung of the ladder. My job included admitting patients who were there for routine surgery and undertaking accompanied ward rounds with the consultant and registrar, gathering a list of tasks for each patient on the way round which then kept me busy for most of the rest of the day. I also took part in the on-call rota with two other doctors of the same junior standing, so had to be on-call for evenings and weekends. However, the out of hours workload was less than in any other job that I did, apart from psychiatry, so it was not too onerous. Emergency calls seemed to be either severe nosebleeds that needed cautery or packing, or both, and foreign objects stuck in the throat. Most commonly and notably these would be fish bones. I could not remember a single Friday on-call when I did not have to deal with at least one these latter incidents. Of course, one had to remain vigilant. Whilst it may well be that the commonest cause of nose bleeds is long fingernails, there is always the chance that the patient has a serious underlying medical condition that has affected the clotting ability of the blood, and we picked up cases of liver disease and leukaemia amongst other things, so it was not just a matter of stuffing up nostrils and sending patients on their way. I also had to help in the Outpatient clinics where I would review returning patients for on-going problems, with input from the consultants where necessary, or I would undertake minor procedures in a mini clinic of its own. Of these latter procedures, two in particular have stuck in my memory. The first was with an elderly lady who had a chronic inflammatory condition that affected the nose (and other organs around the body such as the kidneys and joints) and which over the years had caused significant nasal tissue destruction and had resulted in deformity of the nasal architecture and a chronic infection. This poor lady had to attend clinic every few months to have a junior doctor slowly peel away the accumulated scab from the whole of the inside of her nose, and deal with the underlying pus to leave her with a reasonably clear nasal airway for a while and to remove the smell that she experienced from this putrefaction with every breath in. The periodicity was such that she must have had a different doctor each time, for these junior training posts lasted six months at a time, and thus none was particularly adept at the process, which must have been extremely unpleasant for the patient. Of course, it was not a barrel of laughs for the doctor either, and I hoped that I maintained a reasonable poker face and that my distaste for the task did not show too much. At least I knew that I would not have to do it a second time. The other memorable procedure was one regularly performed for patients suffering with chronic sinusitis. The human body is not well designed for upright living in many ways, and the drainage of the sinuses is one such design flaw. The drainage holes for the maxillary sinuses, the main sinus in the cheeks, lie above the floor of the hollow area when a person stands upright, which explains why these sinuses often drain better if somebody bends over forwards and thus re-orientates the drainage hole to the lowest point. Therefore, with a chronic sinus infection there is the possibility that this area below the drainage hole forms a sump which collects pus and debris and makes life for the sufferer miserable. These days, endoscopic surgery, and lavage, or rinsing, are used, but back then it was my job to drain these as an outpatient procedure under local anaesthetic. The idea was to numb the area on the lateral (or outside) wall of the nasal cavity just where the bone was thinnest. The way this was done was to use cocaine paste, for cocaine is a highly effective local anaesthetic. Long thin sticks of wood, like lollipop sticks, had cotton wool wound around the top to form an elongated cotton bud, and then paste was applied to the cotton wool and this was inserted in the nose under the turbinate bone on the lateral wall. The turbinate is a cylindrical bone that runs the length of the nasal cavity and is covered in a mucosal lining with a rich blood supply to moisten and warm the air as it makes its way through the nose *en route* to the respiratory tract. There are three such bones on each side and the lower two are easily visible from the nostril. The sticks with the paste on sat just under the lowest turbinate on each side. There were usually several cases to do and so there was eventually a short row of patients sitting in the corridor in outpatients, each with a wooden stick protruding from their nostril on one or both sides. Obviously, cocaine has other effects when administered via the nose, and there would always be at least one patient who was more susceptible to its soporific effect, possibly because it was impossible to dose the amount via the paste used. I presume that those who use the drug recreationally are similarly plagued by problems of inconsistent dosage and unpredictable response. Therefore, those patients who were affected would feel light-headed and faint, although a little carefree too, and then had to be laid down and watched over by one of the nurses. Once the numbing effect was sufficient, I had to take each patient in turn into a side room, get them resting back comfortably on a couch, remove the stick and its coating of medicament, and then use a trocar and cannula to punch through the bone from the nasal cavity and into the offending sinus. The cannula is a metal tube and it contained the trocar which is a sturdy metal point that fitted snugly inside the tube with the point protruding from the end. The point was placed under the turbinate bone once the improvised cotton bud had been removed, and gentle but sustained pressure was applied. The bone was paper thin here, but still made a slightly sickening crunch as it gave way, which must have been unpleasant for the patient concerned, even though they could feel nothing. Then the trocar was withdrawn, and syringefuls of warm salty water were used to irrigate the sinuses in turn via the cannula until the liquid running out each time was clear. If this procedure had to be repeated, it was easier to do but less likely to be effective and then the patient faced more definitive surgery to produce a permanent draining aperture. Once the cannula was removed after the lavage procedure it left a handy drainage hole for the sinus, until the nasal lining healed and sealed it up again.

This was not a procedure that I ever needed in Primary Care, but I did learn another that was useful on several occasions, which was the drainage of a quinsy. For those who do not know, a quinsy is not an American drama from the 1970s about a medical examiner who sports a face like a bloodhound with a hangover and scores an unlikely success rate with the ladies but is a retro-tonsillar abscess. This is usually a complication of acute bacterial tonsillitis, and if you thought that tonsillitis made you feel sick, then just try having a quinsy. The retro-tonsillar space is small and the pressure of the build-up of pus there is very painful, apart from the toxic effects of the infection. The way that I learned to deal with this was to aspirate it with a needle and syringe. Firstly, the patient was laid down so that they could not back their head away. I have yet to meet a patient who will willing advance towards a needle and syringe heading for their mouth. And these were big needles and syringes. The needle needed a decent calibre to make a hole into the abscess areas through the soft palate from which any residual pus could drain after the aspiration. This needle was attached to a 20 ml syringe, not because of the expectation of this volume of pus, but because the 20ml size is of robust plastic and long enough to ensure that I could withdraw the plunger from beyond the patient's incisor teeth. If they bit down mid-procedure then they would bite onto the syringe, which was robust enough to take it, and not my fingers. We used our old friendly local anaesthetic cocaine again, this time as a spray, to numb the soft palate before the procedure. I often wondered later just how much cocaine was used in the ENT department and just how it was kept logged, as quantities such as "one spray" seemed hopelessly inaccurate. Anyway, it did the job and then I could advance with my needle and syringe into the mouth cavity. Once the needle had entered the anaesthetised palate, I drew back on the plunger of the syringe, whilst slowly advancing the needle until I hit paydirt and two or three millilitres of turbid pus was drawn back into the barrel. At that point I withdrew, followed by a small gush of blood from the palate and large gush of gratitude from the patient who felt immediately better, notwithstanding the on-going tonsillitis that would usually respond to antibiotics. I undertook this procedure several times in Primary Care, once to the horror of the senior partner in my first practice who watched me and claimed he "wouldn't do that in a fit!" However, this procedure, like so many, has fallen foul of the cautious approaches of the medicolegal indemnity companies, whose attitude always struck me as being like that of Sergeant Wilson from Dad's Army, who would respond to the impulsive and daring ideas of his superior, Captain Mainwaring, with the line "Are you sure that is wise?" These days, seemingly, very little is any more.

The other thing about ENT was that it finally showed me just what that ring-shaped appendage was that was often depicted on the forehead of doctors whenever the image of one was shown. It was, in fact, a mirror, which was concave so that it focussed light, and with a central hole such that it resembled a shiny ring doughnut. It would be strapped to the forehead of the doctor so that it could be swung down over one eye and they could look through the hole. Then, a lamp placed behind the seated patient was switched on so that it shone onto the mirror, and the light from that lamp was focussed by the concavity and reflected onto whatever the doctor was looking directly at with the eye over which the mirror was positioned. This enabled the doctor to illuminate the throat or nose that they were examining whilst leaving both hands free to use other implements to improve the view. When looking at the voice box, or larynx, an angled mirror on a long handle was used and was held against the soft palate at the back of the throat, to prevent the dangling uvula there from obscuring the view. Of course, the patient's breath was warmer than the mirror and so the reflective surface would usually have instantly misted up from the moisture in the breath condensing on it. Therefore, it had to be first gently warmed by being held briefly over a small glass desk-top paraffin burner, with a wick and small receptacle for the purple paraffin beneath, and which looked exactly like the scented oil burners that became popular in homes some twenty years later. This warming of the mirror prevented the condensation forming and allowed a view of the larynx working as the patient followed instructions to make certain vocal sounds. This was always provided that the inexperienced doctor had not over-warmed the metal mirror over the flame, thus risking burning the patient's soft palate, or did not press too hard at the back of the throat with the mirror, thus triggering the gag reflex and risking a lap full of the patient's last meal. Thankfully, these contraptions have now been consigned to history and replaced by a small fibre-optic endoscope that is passed in through a nostril and can be bent once above the soft palate, to enable the operator to look straight down at the larynx from above and give a much clearer view than I ever had. However, this by-gone age of medicine is really not so long ago in the past.

The next job was in Rheumatology, which encompassed all types of arthritis and their medical, but not surgical treatment. The latter aspect formed part of Orthopaedic Surgery, which was a speciality I did not undertake. I found Rheumatology to be fascinating as most of the conditions involved many organs of the body, it was just that the most obvious manifestation of the disease was in the joints, causing pain and stiffness and loss of function. Many treatments at the time had not developed much from the early part of the twentieth century, and some patients still received mediaeval sounding treatments such as injections of gold for their Rheumatoid Arthritis. Such treatments have long since been superseded by therapies which much more specifically target the inflammatory process that causes the damage. Aspirin-based anti-inflammatory medications and steroids, administered both by mouth and injection, were also commonly used treatments and remain so to this day. The job was a good grounding for holistic patient assessment and the understanding of a multiplicity of symptoms and interested me to such an extent that I seriously considered a change in career direction at this point, supported by the senior consultant there at the time. Finally, I decided to stay on the track I had taken but was able to apply this new learning to the many patients with joint problems that I saw in General Practice subsequently.

I also learned to be careful with my questioning. One of the cardinal symptoms of joint inflammation is that joints feel stiff on first use after a period of inactivity, easing with use, and then stiffening up again after further rest. However, asking one elderly gentleman if he got much morning stiffness he replied that the "old fella" was not as active as it used to be in his youth, much to his regret. I then had to point out that I was asking about his joint health rather than his erectile potency and resolved to rephrase the question in future.

The job involved two three-month elements on rotation with another clinician, with the first three months in the main hospital in Norwich, but the second three months split between two peripheral hospitals. One of these was in the market town of Aylsham and the establishment bore all the hallmarks of an old-style small community hospital, albeit with the latest equipment at the time. There were wards and small operating theatres, outpatient clinics, and a pleasing campus of grounds in which the hospital sat, with staff accommodation on site and close by, with the whole overseen by a large and benevolent-looking water tower. The other establishment was on the north-east Norfolk coast and had once been a hospital for consumptive patients back in the day. Built with a mock-Tudor I, it had a long veranda on the sea-ward side, which in my time still held several substantial wooden seats that had sides and a roof but were open at the front and could be pivoted in any direction. The patient suffering from consumption would previously have been ensconced in one of these, wrapped up in many layers of clothing against the biting cold, and the seat would be turned to face the icy wind as it swept across the North Sea from the Urals, all in the hope that it would overwhelm the infection with a blast of the freshest of air. These poor souls had little else in the way of treatment that could be offered to them. The key role of this rheumatological outpost these days was to help rehabilitate patients suffering from the significant joint disruption and damage caused by the arthritic disease process which the treatments of the day only partially addressed, or for rehabilitation after joint replacement surgery. The medications used these days affect the disease process so much that such damage to the joints is rarely seen. The rehabilitative role of the hospital meant that the Physiotherapists and Occupational Therapists were kept busy all the time, whereas there were no acute admissions or clinics here, and I had little to do after completing the tasks that had been highlighted in the morning ward round with the consultant other than be available should there be a collapse or other such emergency. I did do some studying, of course, but I also drank a lot of coffee and played the odd frame of snooker on the old full-sized slate-based table that lay quietly under its cover down in the bowels of the hospital and was seemingly almost forgotten if the dust on the cue rack and table covering were anything to go by. I never worked out if the table was intended as part of the patient's rehabilitation or was there for the amusement of resident staff, but I never saw evidence of anyone else using it.

Sadly, both medical outposts are no more. The coastal one was sold into the hands of a private mental health clinic which unfortunately fell afoul of the Care Quality Commission and had to close, and the other was closed to have some of the grounds sold off for private housing, whilst the main hospital building itself was converted into a care home.

The job in psychiatry was at an acute unit at a site in Norwich, rather than any of the several outlying ones that were around at the time and have since closed, and the patients were there voluntarily for the most part. I have alluded to the habitual dress of the staff so that they did not stand out too much against their charges. They also had a communal breakfast with the team report meeting each morning, and they all seemed to smoke like chimneys. The on-call duty was not too onerous, and I usually slept soundly in one of the small on-call rooms with high ceilings and draughty sash windows to be found in the Victorian era block on site. The windows also rattled with the slightest breeze, and I was unfortunate enough to be on-call on the night of the hurricane in 1987 so there was no sleep that night. I also had to stay longer as the way home was blocked by fallen trees. This was probably the most noteworthy event of the whole six months, but I got a lot of valuable experience.

CHAPTER 10

The last hospital job on my rotation was in Paediatrics. I did this job in a hospital near the coast, rather than the main one in Norwich previously referred to, and I got this job at the second attempt. I had applied a few years earlier, but been turned down, though I was given feed-back at the time suggesting that I should try again when I had more experience under my belt. This seemed reasonable once I eventually got a job there two years later, as the hospital did not have the full range of support and departmental backup that the larger District General Hospital enjoyed. In this role I dealt with acute admissions to the wards from GPs and via Accident and Emergency, planned admissions for treatment to chronic conditions, and I helped with outpatient clinics. The job was made easier as I had experience with my own children by then too, and I conceded that this might have been part of what was meant at my first interview. I certainly noticed a difference with one of my colleagues who did not have children. One of the daily morning jobs for the senior house officers was to do the rounds of the post-natal wards to do medical checks on any new babies that had been born overnight. All such babies have a comprehensive check within twenty-four hours of birth to look at the major systems in the body for problems that might not have been picked up during ante-natal scans, and to ensure that the usual physiological changes that occur in babies after birth had satisfactorily occurred. For example, there are major changes in a baby's circulation once it goes from getting all its oxygen supply from the mother's circulation via the placenta, to getting it from the ambient air via its own lungs instead. These checks included checking the genitalia for abnormalities in case there was gender uncertainty, checking the hips for a full range of movement in case there is any hip dysplasia or postural problem from the orientation of the baby in the womb, checking the anus for perforation, listening to the heart sounds and the air entry into the lungs, and palpating the major pulses in the groin to exclude the possibility of a narrowing of the aorta, which is the main artery from the left side of the heart. Naturally, some of these checks involved removing the nappy, and it was common to find that baby had marked its first night in the outside world by the passage of material from the back passage, such material being called meconium at this stage rather than stool. Upon finding a nappy thus soiled, I just used the front of the nappy to clear the majority, finished my checks, and passed the baby back to its mother or a midwife for a more comprehensive dealing with the matter in hand. My colleague, on first finding this unpleasant material lurking within the nappy he was removing, recoiled in horror, and immediately called out "Help, help, midwife emergency, this child's done a poo!" This call was usually met with much tutting and rolling upwards of the eyes by the midwives on the ward who were already busy enough. Sometimes though, his helplessness would engender sympathy and a fussing around to get things done for him, whereas I would get no such support or help. If you looked like you could cope, you were generally left to get on with it and this was a situation that I found throughout my experience in the NHS.

Paediatricians were also called to attend deliveries of women where there was some resuscitation of the new-born could be anticipated, such as any instrumental or surgical delivery, and if the mother had received pethidine for pain relief, or if there had been signs of foetal distress either on the monitor trace of the baby's heart-beat, or if distress had been shown by the baby having voided its bowels of meconium which then appeared in the liquor which accompanied them as they emerged from their mother's womb. I would arrive at the site of the action and take charge of a small trolley which had a heater overhead, and a gently sloping surface upon which the new-born would be laid upon a towel, on its back and with its head towards me and at the lowest point of the incline. An assessment of its condition was taken using the APGAR scoring (standing for Appearance,

Pulse, Grimace, Activity and Respiration, each element getting a score between zero and two) and another such was taken at the end of any intervention, before the baby either went back to mother or on to the Special Care Baby Unit (SCBU) for further treatment. If the mother had received pethidine then the baby would need an intramuscular injection of an antidote to it, to prevent the opiate depressing the baby's respiratory function as it would have crossed the placenta into their circulation. This always seemed a particularly harsh introduction to the outside world. They also may need suction of the nose and mouth to clear secretions there. The usual mechanical suction apparatus is too harsh for this job and so the gentler suction of a human mouth is used via a small piece of apparatus which consisted of two tubes connected via a small clear plastic container. The first tube went to the paediatrician's mouth, and the tube extended just beyond the inner surface of the plastic container. The other tube went to the baby and extended further in. The idea was that any material sucked into the container would not go on into the mouth of the operator, and this worked well as long as one got the tubes the right way around. It only took one mouthful of gubbins to double-check thereafter. If they had breathing problems then there was ambient oxygen to apply but they may have then needed intubation if they failed to respond, and they would definitely have then gone on to SCBU instead of back to mum.

I found working SCBU the most difficult. These tiny scraps of humanity had often suffered whilst in the womb from a poor supply of nutrition, or from lack of oxygen whilst in transit to the outside world and were usually then submitted to a dramatic change in environment by being untimely ripped from their mother if an emergency Caesarean section was needed due to their distress *in utero* and they were too fragile to be submitted to the traumas of normal childbirth. They then lay in their incubators, with tubes inserted and wires attached, walking a tightrope of homeostasis as their immature systems struggled to adjust to the challenges of the outside world. They may have looked at ease under their sunbeds, with eye-pads on rather than shades to protect their retinae from ultraviolet light damage, but I knew that this ultraviolet light might be all that was keeping them from poisoning their own system with their bilirubin. This is produced by the breakdown of haemoglobin from red blood cells and is a normal process that is comfortably handled by the liver in most circumstances. However, in the new-born infant there is a surfeit of red blood cells that they had needed in utero because of the lower oxygen saturations available when they were absorbing oxygen from their mother's blood rather than direct from the surrounding air. These foetal cells, with their own specialised form of haemoglobin, were now surplus to requirements, and they were being broken down within the body, releasing their haemoglobin to be metabolised, a process of which bilirubin is an end-product. However, for some babies, their livers were too immature to process this surge of breakdown product into harmless material to be excreted from the body, and thus it accumulated in the skin and elsewhere in the body, potentially with toxic results. The ultraviolet light affects the bilirubin so that it is easier to clear from the body.

I found it traumatic to have to re-site cannulas into these babies, whose veins seemed to be too insubstantial to stand such assault with a metal or plastic tube, however small in calibre. I was fortunate that there was only one death amongst the neonates in the six months that I spent doing that job, and that was hard enough for me to process. Another tough ask was to patiently deal with parents who clearly did not have a clue about how to manage the responsibility of caring for a child. I thought my own children to be the most precious thing in my life, and that I was privileged to be charged with their welfare, so it was difficult to see the results of some parents who did not share that view or who saw their own offspring as an unwelcome distraction from their own immediate gratification, and, therefore, as a nuisance that surely somebody else must be responsible for.

The one thing that all of these diverse jobs had in common was that I received no training in any of them before starting. You just turned up on day one and had to cope. For any specific procedure I would be talked through it once by a registrar, usually in person but occasionally over the phone, and having successfully done it once I was considered safe to fly solo thereafter. This was the medical adage of "See one, Do one, Teach one" that I presume still exists. There was certainly never any spare capacity to allow me to take time off from a current job to be trained in the skills needed for the next one.

One of the things that I deliberately chose not to do during my training, was to study for membership of the Royal College of General Practitioners. This membership is essential now, but was optional then, though it was rapidly gaining in popularity. I felt that, if everybody had this qualification, then it was no way to differentiate between job candidates. Also, having investigated it, I could not afford the fees, let alone the cost of the weekend course that you had to attend to learn the sort of strategy necessary to pass the examination.

An example of such a strategy was a question about how one would approach the care of a child with apparent earache who had been brought into surgery by a fractious mother. The ideal answer would have to include one asking for a full history of birth, pregnancy and childhood up to that point, whether the child had reached appropriate developmental milestones and received its full complement of immunisations against the common infectious diseases, whether there were any other children in the family, and how they were, whether the family was known to Social Services, whether both parents were present at home and what jobs they did, if any, whether they smoked, whether the mother had suffered any mental health problems at any time, and especially during or since the pregnancy, if the child was well nourished and dressed and obviously cared for, why the child had been presented at this particular point and what the parental expectations were, well before consideration of a thorough examination of the child, prescription of any necessary medications, giving advice on how to administer those, and asking after the welfare of the rest of the family. Whilst all of this information is important and highly relevant, to answer a question thus implies that all of this can be achieved in a consultation lasting just five minutes, for it would be another decade before ten-minute appointments became the norm, and of course that is just ridiculous. Even ten minutes is too little to allow for all of that, especially as one would have to then carefully document everything too before moving on to the next patient on the list. Realistically, it might just be that the child had a sore ear, and the mother was fractious because the child had kept her awake all night, but of course nobody would give that answer and expect to pass the exam. The strength of General Practice is that one knows the rest of the family and their circumstances or can easily access that information from notes or a colleague. With experience I also learned to assess mother and child and their interaction very quickly within the first minute or so of any consultation, and to a point where it was almost subliminal. The idea that tactical answering was necessary to gain enough marks to pass this examination just did not make sense to me, and so I decided not to do it. Another aspect of my ASD I suppose. There were numerous certificates and diplomas available as post-graduate qualifications in various specialities and made the post-nominals of many of my contemporaries look more like a sequence in DNA than anything else, but I pursued none of them myself.

Despite this supposed deficit I managed to get jobs throughout my career. The only time lack of membership was a barrier was when I investigated working abroad. I seriously considered a return to the Antipodes to live and work rather than just visit, for the rewards for being GP there were considerably greater than in the NHS, and the potential for a beneficial work-life balance was significantly improved. However, the membership of the Royal College was needed as proof of equivalent training, and a decade or so of appropriate experience was not. Besides, when asked, Rebekah stated that under no circumstances would she be moving to the other side of the world on any account, so I had to defer. By the time the Royal College qualification had become obligatory for newly qualified doctors in their GP training, I had many years of experience to offer any prospective employer which more than compensated for the deficiency in letters after my name. Indeed, the acquisition of letters was of no interest to me, just as I was not particularly bothered about whether people used my correct title when addressing me. Many would consider me to lack ambition, but I just wanted to do the best job that I could and to make a difference to the patients I saw. I had no political or leadership aspirations and found that seeing patients and trying to find out what was wrong with them was endlessly fascinating. I did not feel the need for a large arena in which to do this and, whilst policy and guidance would always need to be formulated by others, I saw my job as dealing with the patient in front of me at any given time, and seeing how, or if, the policy and guidance applied to that patient and their own medical situation. Medical policies and protocols are based upon research evidence, with most patients in a treatment group needing to show benefit from whatever intervention was being assessed. However, within that treatment group there would be individuals who gained no benefit, or were even harmed by the intervention, so I have always seen my job as trying to identify which category the patient sat in front of me belonged to and acting accordingly. Although evidence-based medicine is the gold standard these days, it must be remembered that the evidence only shows benefit for the majority, not for everybody.

CHAPTER 11

Rebekah and I married quite early into my GP training rotation, mostly because she was keen to do so, and I could not think of a suitable reason to delay. We had a rocky time (no pun intended) because of the separation when I had been away in Gibraltar, but the relationship survived that separation and we seemed and felt secure together. We had bought our first home and I felt that I was settling into my career and environment. Rebekah's family welcomed me, and I was at home in their company. It was only much later that I learned that the same could not be said of my family's attitude towards Rebekah. They did not share that opinion with me, however, and felt that they should do their best to tolerate Rebekah with a good grace for my sake. Time would show that their concerns about our suitability were well founded but they never admonished me for not taking heed of the reticence that they had shown.

I had made few friends and brought none with me, so our social life revolved around Rebekah's social circle as she had been born and raised in Norfolk and many family members and school friends were still in the area. Indeed, we seemed to be unable to leave the house without seeing somebody that she had known "forever", and it became a standing joke with us wherever we went, home or abroad, as to whom we might run into that she knew. The journey to Kent from Norfolk was long, and free time was in short supply, and the trips to see my family became less frequent and became replaced by weekly phone calls. I was complicit in this as I got rather fed up with my mother's comments of how tired I looked whenever she saw me, and her expressed view that I should just work a little less, and she simply did not seem to understand the work pressures that I faced. There was no option of "downing tools" at "knocking off time" – these concepts simply did not exist in my chosen field. Indeed, I never got a dedicated meal break of any sort for the

duration of my career. When in hospital, food was grabbed on the run from the canteen or a vending machine or was possibly just a handful of chocolates
or biscuits from the supply left at the nurses' station by a grateful patient at whichever ward I was on at the time. In Primary Care, lunch was something packed and eaten in the car between home visits or at my desk whilst poring over letters and pathology results or the actions arising from them, or signing piles of prescriptions, or dictating letters, or requesting tests, or responding to queries, or any number of other things. My mother seemed unable to comprehend the workload and responsibility of my profession and I got tired of repeatedly trying to explain and excuse it. Dad's response was usually that she should "leave the boy alone" but that made no real contribution to either side. However, Rebekah did little to help improve the situation or welcome my family. My parents came up to see us from time to time but had to stay in a guest house as Rebekah pointedly refused to give up her bed to accommodate them or, when we had moved and had a family of our own and a bigger house, to compel any of the children to do so.
It was only three months after our wedding that Rebekah started to feel a bit unwell, and tests showed her to be pregnant. She had been taking precautions, or so she told me, and there had been no discussion about starting a family so soon, but there was never any suggestion of her not continuing the pregnancy. This turned out to be just as well because, although we eventually had three children, these were interspersed with several miscarriages and a molar pregnancy and so, not only were the children precious, but they were also hard won.
I set about married life with a will. I never looked for more and, throughout the years that followed, my home and family were the centre of my world. I decorated the bungalow throughout, re-laid and enlarged the small patio in the south-facing back garden and changed the planting in the garden from the inherited palate of green and gold evergreen heathers and conifers to deciduous and fruiting bushes and shrubs so that

the wildlife did not find it quite such a barren wasteland. There was a huge leylandii hedge at the foot of the garden which was already too tall and wide to manage when we moved in. I tussled with it over the few years we were there, with it trying to block out the sunshine from the whole garden, and me trying to keep it down to a vaguely manageable height and depth using only rudimentary tools and a wobbly stepladder, but it still seemed to both dominate and slowly erode the garden space.

Rose, our first child, duly arrived on her expected date, one of the few times in her childhood when she was punctual, and she was established into the back bedroom of the bungalow which I had decorated out as a nursery. It had been Rebekah and my bedroom, but we decided to move into the front to leave the warmer and brighter room for Rose. By that time, we also had a dog, Smidge, a small terrier who was affectionate and well behaved, if you discounted the two wallets of mine that he had thoroughly chewed when a puppy, and the hall carpet that he scrapped up into a tangle of threads and a debris of backing felt when he was left in the hall but wanted to get into the lounge and thus tried to dig his way through. He was black and white with a fringed tail and roguish disposition and walking him was one extra chore that I really did not need in my already-busy schedule. However, I was aware that he was company for Rebekah whilst I was away on-call in the hospital several nights per week, and so I did not feel I could begrudge her that.

I was still working through the succession of jobs that I needed to complete for my General Practitioner training, which meant yet more nights and weekends away from home whilst on duty in the various hospitals. I appreciated that this left Rebekah to manage alone, hence the reason for the dog as mentioned, but night-time duties at home still fell to me when I was there regardless of my recent on-call experiences or the need to be up early the following day for work. Rebekah considered my nights at home to be her nights off and made sure I completely understood that. Therefore, I never really got a night off for twenty years, and I walked the dog every morning that I was at home. If I was not at home, the dog missed out. I needed the car for the commute to work and so Rebekah was a little isolated out on the edge of the broads in those early days. Money was tight, for her income had dropped, we had borrowed all we could for that first mortgage, and a second car was simply not affordable. However, there then came a time when I needed to undertake the job in paediatrics on the coast. It was for the six months heading into Winter, the journey times were longer, and Rebekah would potentially be isolated at home for days at a time when I was on-call, and so it was felt that a second car had become a necessity.

Our budget was severely limited, which, in turn, limited our options. I therefore searched the "jalopy for sale" column in the back of the local paper looking for cars with a service history and a reasonable MOT remaining that might get us through until later in the year at least. Eventually I spotted an advertisement for an old Vauxhall Viva for sale which had nine remaining months on its MOT, and which cost the princely sum of £150. It was for sale up on the coast, near to the old rehabilitation hospital I had worked in for Rheumatology. So, we drove up to the Norfolk coast to locate the seller who lived behind a row of old farm cottages in one of the many villages there. On first inspection, and even without much mechanical knowledge I could immediately see that this car was unlikely to pass another MOT. The advertisement had declared the car to be "in need of some welding," but this description understated by some degree the level of disintegration of the floor of the driver and front passenger foot wells. It seemed as if it were only the integrity of the carpet laid there that prevented the drivers' feet from reaching the road, in the manner of the Flintstone vehicles from the cartoons that I remembered from my childhood and would be subsequently reminded of through the viewing habits of my own children.

Despite its apparent limitations regarding structural integrity, the car started on the first turn despite a cold engine, and it idled nicely and sounded OK when the accelerator was pressed.

There was a large yard behind the cottages, so a test drive was possible. There was a slight grinding sound when driving the car in reverse gear, but the gearbox was otherwise nice and smooth. The wipers worked, as did all the lights, and the exhaust was not blowing. It looked a bit odd, mostly because no two adjacent body panels of the car seemed to be the exact shade of yellow as each other, but that was just cosmetics. The inside blower worked, but produced only chilly air, even, I later found, when the engine had been running a while and thus had warmed up nicely. Even on full blast it was certainly not man enough to clear the condensation from the inside of the windscreen that had accumulated from the high moisture content of the carpets on the floor, so it was more like a sound effect than a useful bit of apparatus. A cloth or towel was needed to wipe the inside surface of the screen instead, and in all weathers, although when it became warmer the windows could be left open to create a through draft and this also helped.

Therefore, I parted with my cash and brought the car home. Despite the apparent problems with it, the basic machinery proved sound enough and it successfully carried me back and forth to the coastal job throughout the six-month term that I was there, all through the winter weather, continuing to start first go and grind in reverse, but secure and sturdy. True, I could have done with brighter headlights, especially on dark mornings when the snow was coming down and was being driven towards me by an icy Easterly wind, but it coped. In fact, it continued to run well until just before the nine-month term of the MOT was up, when all major parts and the engine seized at once and it went from being a "good little runner" to an accumulation of scrap metal, without passing through any intermediate stage. But it had done its job and was fondly remembered, by me at least. Rebekah, who would never dare set foot in it even as a passenger, had always referred to it as "The Pineapple Prat-mobile," but seemed happy enough for me to be driving it. By the time its race was run, our finances had improved a little and a second car was duly purchased for

Rebekah's regular use, something a little newer and considerably more robust than the Viva had been.

I had now gone through all of my hospital training jobs and had arrived at the stage of doing my final six-month stint as a GP trainee, after which I could apply to be considered a GP on the Performer's List and seek a position in a practice of my own. I got some idea of the world of General Practice in this placement, though the grounding I received fell below the level of training I should have got regarding exactly what being a partner entailed. The idea of being a trainee in a practice was that I was meant to be supernumerary, and the practice was paid by the deanery to accommodate me, so that I had more time with patients and could spend time discussing any problems with my supervisor, who was the senior partner in the practice. Instead, my workload in this practice was the same as all of the partners, and I got little or no protected time for the training element. All that the supervising partner did was give me video tapes of medical issues to watch. When I took holiday, the practice was forced to employ a locum to cover my absence, which should never have been needed if I was supernumerary. It appeared that the practice took on trainee GPs to provide an extra pair of hands whilst getting paid by the Deanery at the same time, whereas what they really needed was an extra partner. They certainly did very well out of the arrangement as it gave them an easier time, at no cost to themselves. Given some of my later experiences, this introduction to the mercenary attitude of some GPs turned out to be an appropriate training opportunity after all. Once I was signed off at the end of this job I was at last free at last to pursue my own career path, but I was to find it a bumpier road than I had imagined.

CHAPTER 12

Believe it or not given the current climate, in the 1980s becoming a General Practitioner in the UK was an extremely popular career choice for doctors. Incomes were good, workload was manageable, and, despite all surgeries covering their own patients on-call over-nights and at weekends, patients were less inclined to call their doctor out after surgery closed. GP surgeries reported no shortage of doctors wishing to become partners, and there were often twenty or more applications for every vacancy that was advertised thus competition was fierce. However, I was not daunted by this and made several applications to vacancies in practices in the local area and was lucky that I was offered a partnership within three months of qualifying as an independent practitioner. I spent this time working as a short-term locum in a variety of different settings, covering doctors who were absent on leave or through illness. I had decided that I would only apply to vacant positions in more rural locations as I had worked in both a rural and a suburban practice in my training, and I much preferred the former. Although the practice area was likely to be much larger, and the patients could be wide-spread and isolated, meaning more time spent on the road and less accessible support and help if required, I found it a much more pleasant working environment. There was also a more intrepid feel to working in those situations. During my first training post near the Norfolk Broads, I had spent some interesting nights trying to find patients in dark cottages down unmade roads or overgrown lanes, as well as temporary patients who had come there on holiday, only to fall ill and require the local doctor to be called out. Patients who came away without their asthma inhalers, only to suffer an attack in an unfamiliar environment were a particular theme, made more taxing by the lack of electricity with which to run the nebuliser in some locations. The practice had owned an ancient foot-operated nebuliser and I had spent several wet nights on various moored holiday craft administering to patients caught out in this way. It was all valuable experience.

The practice I joined was in the middle of a rural triangle, at each angle of which was a large market town, each having one or two GP practices of their own. This practice had four partners, including myself, and they were spread over two premises. I should have spotted potential problems then really, as it was difficult to determine if either was a branch surgery or not. Historically, the "main" surgery belonged to a practice where there had previously been a husband-and-wife partnership who had been there for decades, and the tales from that time showed both extremes of what rural General Practice had been like, back in the day. There were many tales of how the husband in the partnership would never let work get in the way of real life, and how communication could be tenuous at best in those days before mobile phones were even dreamed of, and not every home had a landline. There were stories, possibly apocryphal but, I felt, probably not, of how this doctor would leave notes on his front door for anybody wishing to contact him in an emergency, such as "gone fishing up-stream" or "bell-ringing practice," or even just "gone out" with some rough approximation of the time of his return. Patients were then expected to track him down to request his attention and hopefully drag him away from whatever he was doing at the time. The other extreme was the behaviour of his wife, who could clearly only cope with the demands of the life they had chosen by blotting out the reality of it with copious amounts of alcohol, and she subsequently developed cirrhosis of the liver as a result. Of the two, despite them both having long careers, it was she who bowed out first, from the work at the practice initially, and then existence entirely.

The origin of the other surgery at the practice was that a single-handed GP had retired after serving that community alone for many years, and his practice area abutted that of the husband-

and-wife team. The two partners at the first surgery had decided to approach the new incumbent at the second with a view to them joining forces, presumably because a rota of one in three nights and weekends on call was better than either a one in two, or being on-call every night and weekend, depending on who you were. Unfortunately, this amalgamation seems to have been an uneasy affair despite both surgeries implying that they would be equal, as the two partners at one end rather assumed that they were the main practice, and the former single-handed one was the branch, much to the chagrin of the doctor at this end who did not feel that he had agreed to become subservient to them having previously run his own practice alone. Beneath the surface bonhomie, all was clearly not well within the partnership, and they tried to patch this up with the idea of getting a fourth partner who could work at both surgeries, thus linking them more effectively, and providing a fourth doctor to share the rota. This was the partnership that I took on, whilst unwittingly becoming the glue that it was hoped would help make a functioning whole from the disparate constituent parts. There was certainly no sign of friction during the interview process and visits to the buildings, or chats with the staff. Unfortunately for all concerned, underlying frictions did not take too long to become apparent. Far from joining both surgeries together, I felt that I was a part of neither and, as such, a friend and confidante of neither of the two warring factions, so my professional life was a constant compromise. I also felt that I was being made the butt of anything that went wrong. After a few years, the senior partner, who worked at the two-handed end, left the practice to rush back to his native Antipodes, actively pursued by the tax man after a business venture collapsed, and a new partner was taken on to replace him. He was something of a manipulator and worked his way in nicely, so that I got the impression the other three partners met together and decided on strategy before we had formal partners meetings, as ideas and plans always came to the meetings fully formed and with three votes behind them. I therefore had no real say in anything despite being a full business partner in the practice.

I put up with this for a dozen years, but then decided I had been the whipping boy without any say for long enough, and so I walked away. The idea of a principal leaving a partnership was almost unheard of at the time when the tendency was more towards sticking it out to the grim death, with worsening relations. Partially this was because there was still competition for jobs, and a partner who left was somehow seen as tainted. After all, who could I use as referees other than my former partners, and if relations were sour what sort of reference would they give, both on and off the record? There were many stories from various practices where partners had decided to dig in and stick it out, but where the feuds became ingrained and obvious in that they simply refused to acknowledge each other's existence, let alone share a cup of coffee together. This ended up with them effectively working in silos with no practice-wide view of anything and no chance for professional consultation or communication, which can only have been to the detriment of patient care. It must also have been an exceedingly difficult place to work for all of the other staff, who would constantly be walking on eggshells or having to act as intermediaries between the warring parties.

I felt I had given it every chance to work, but eventually conceded that it had not, and could not do so. When I left I did not get so much as a good luck card from my professional partners. I had definitely made the right decision.

Within a very few years of my leaving that practice, all of the other partners had also left, two of them to move abroad, and one who left General Practice entirely to work for the Care Quality Commission. Perhaps I had been the lynchpin that kept things together because the whole house of cards tumbled once I had left. I therefore looked for an alternative practice. In this, I had even more restrictions to deal with, as Rebekah flatly refused to move home or her work as a practice nurse. Although she was only working there for two days per week, whilst I was full time, she would not budge on this, as with so many things. Therefore, I was forced to seek a vacancy in a practice in the same area as we lived, which severely limited my options. Fortunately, after some eight months of searching, I did find one and was taken on. I had done a lot of extra out-of-hours work in the region over the years and so both me and my work were known to other GPs in the area, and the need for professional referees was therefore not so great.

I was the second of two partners in this new practice, with me replacing a partner who had retired early due to ill-health. At least I felt that I would have an equal say in things in this practice, which was technically true, and this arrangement worked very well right up until I had a different opinion to that of the incumbent partner. This new partner was fine as long as you agreed with him, but if you did not then the teddies were thrown out of the pram. Initially, I had gone along with the flow of things whilst I was settling in and working my probation period, but it became clear that the practice, whilst in relatively new premises and reasonably profitable, was stagnating and there were changes and developments and investment needed urgently. That was when my new partner showed his true colours, and the reasons why he had been divorced three times and had numerous failed relationships behind him became apparent. He would not discuss, he would not negotiate, he would not compromise, he just wanted his way and was used to getting it. He would take any action, however contradictory, to get his own way in any given situation and would not consider the consequences of his actions. It had turned out to be a case of "out of the frying pan, and into the fire," and I found myself now with the same personality type to deal with at work as I did at home where somebody wanted what they wanted and would consider no alternative. If this was because of the Universe testing me, then I felt it had a warped sense of humour. The worst of it came when my father was in his final days, a combination of prostate cancer and heart failure finally proving more than he could cope with. My partner and I worked four days each week and had a day off each. I would be the duty doctor for Monday and Tuesday, and then have Wednesday off and be the non-duty doctor on a Thursday, when I often tutored medical students in the practice so could not also be on-call. My practice partner had Tuesdays off and was duty doctor on Wednesday and Thursday, and we took turns to be duty doctor on Fridays. Dad was in his final hours and on a syringe driver one Monday, so I asked my partner if he would mind taking over the Tuesday duty so that I could travel down to Kent that night to see my father before he died. My partner refused, saying that he wanted to take his young son to school. I pointed out that he did that every Tuesday whereas this would be my only chance to bid a final farewell to my father, but the partner refused. In fact, he did not show much compassion to anybody else either. I did not want to leave the surgery without medical cover, and I did not feel I could realistically travel after a long duty day, stay up all night in Kent, and travel back again in time for another long duty day, so I aimed to go on the Tuesday evening and hoped that Dad would make it that long. He did not, and I never forgave my partner for robbing me of that opportunity to say goodbye properly. Although I went down as planned the following day, kissing a final goodbye to a cold dead body brought out of the refrigerator for the purpose was not the same as a proper farewell whilst he was alive, even if he would not have been aware of my presence. There were also several things that I would have liked to say to him whilst he was still alive. Suffice to say that this was not what I wanted as a final memory of my father.

CHAPTER 13

Rebekah and I had looked for somewhere to move to once I seemed settled in my first practice, but I had seen how patients would call at the other partner's homes at any time of day or night just because they lived locally and thus were available, and I preferred a bit more privacy when off–duty. Therefore, I chose to live just outside the practice area so that we were not living amongst patients registered to the surgery, but the area was accessible if I was called out at night. Beyond that, we probably did it all wrong really. We did not research schools, or transport links, or think about anything much other than finding a nice house we both liked. I wanted to call it "Bedside Manor" as I liked the pun involved, but in this, like so much else, I was over-ruled. So how did one person over-rule the other you may ask? It was by complicity of course. Although I started out by fighting my corner in what I felt were the sort of negotiations any two people in a relationship would undertake, I forgot that it takes two to negotiate, and the other person must be willing to give ground or compromise in order to come to an agreement. I eventually just allowed it to happen because I had learned that to argue my case was a useless exercise, for Rebekah would never agree to anything other than what she wanted and was immune to any argument, no matter how persuasive or self-evident. In the end I simply could not face having to argue about absolutely everything. I felt I had enough to manage at work without all that aggravation at home. I don't even think that my compliance helped the situation. It merely confirmed to Rebekah that she must have been right all along and thus reinforce in her the belief that her own opinion was the one that mattered most. Also, the consequences for any action were inevitably financial to a degree, and she did not have to fund them. Indeed, she seemed to have no appreciation of money and cost at all, and just spent at will in the expectation that I would cover any shortfall. She once said that her motto in marriage was "What is yours is mine, but what is mine is my own" and that is how she approached things. She kept her wages and the child allowance for her own expenditure and expected me to fund the mortgage, our cars, household expenses, school fees, holidays, and everything else. If she overspent on her income then she just dipped into the household account and complained to me when there was not enough left for food, so that I had to top it up further.

The house we both chose was not quite a ruin, but boy did it need some work. It had stood empty for a while, but we both got a good feeling about it when we viewed it, and both felt that we wanted to live there before either of us mentioned this to the other. At least this was something that we had agreed upon. The original cottage had been built in or around the sixteenth century with a brick base, no true foundations or damp course to speak of, and with the base plate surmounted by a timber frame with wattle and daub infill, or "sticks and shit" as I referred to it. The whole cottage had been built around a substantial brick fireplace and chimney breast with an impressive oak Bessemer beam acting as lintel across the hearth, and consisted of two large rooms, one over the other, comprising the lounge downstairs, and bedroom upstairs. Beyond the chimney was a smaller room which had become the entrance hall, with the space above being part of the landing. To that original building, in the 1970s, had been attached an extension, which comprised a dining room with a second bedroom over it, a kitchen and utility room with a cloakroom off it downstairs, with another bedroom and a family bathroom over them. The whole thing had then been covered in a stippled rendering, no doubt to disguise the blocks used to build the extension and somehow try to meld the old with the new.

The house sat as an island in a small sea of shingle, towards the front boundary of a one-acre paddock which was surrounded by a post-and-rail fence, and which had a two-acre paddock adjoining it. The house was shielded from the road by a mature mixed hedge. The two paddocks were divided by another post-and-rail fence and there was a massive ash tree growing beside the gate between them. Along the road frontage, a little to the side of the cottage and inside the front hedge, was a range of ramshackle outbuildings where the presence of mangers and tethering rings on the wall showed their previous equestrian usage. Whilst the cottage roof was as straight and level as the Fens, that of the outbuildings had an undulating ridge line more reminiscent of the silhouette of the South Downs, and which suggested both extreme age and woodworm. However, the conflicting mechanical forces that were at play within the roof structure seemed to have come to a truce some time ago and there was no sign of instability within it, and it was surprisingly watertight. In this respect it was far superior to the roof of the house itself, though the lack of guttering on the outbuildings led to significant water damage to the brick baseplate from splashing when rain hit the ground instead of being directed away and down a pipe as guttering would have allowed. The outbuildings had a log store at the end, and this was interesting as it contained not only a small quantity of split logs, but also some others that were in a small room off the main store and were intact. Each measured some two to three feet long and bore the vestiges of corrugated paper around them in places. On turning them for closer inspection, I discovered that each of these short logs had the image of what I took to be an African face carved into them. There were male and female represented, and each face was in repose with closed eyes and a calm demeanour. Curiously, they exuded the exact feeling that I felt I perceived about the house itself, and which was one of the things I liked about it. I turned the logs back as I had found them and left them alone. However, a short while later upon returning to the outbuildings, I found that the doorframe to this small compartment had shifted, as evidenced by the lump of wattle and daub that now lay on the floor beneath a deficit in the wall above the low doorway, and the door was now jammed shut. Of course, it could have occurred because I had gone through a doorway that had not been used for some time, but I couldn't help the feeling that perhaps the logs preferred to be left in peace, and so I did just that for the length of our ownership of the property.

At the back of the smaller paddock, just beyond the obligatory post-and-rail fence, was a redundant parish church, whose bells had fallen silent some decades previously. Although it was boarded up, with an overgrown churchyard surrounding it and raucous gang of corvines inhabiting the tower via the louvred apertures through which the sound of the bells would formally have been heard, we found its presence to be dignified and calming, rather than brooding and sinister

Whilst the house had not been lived in, or apparently loved, for some time it still felt like it could be home. For some reason, this unprepossessing house struck a chord with both Rebekah and I at the same time, although each of us felt that the other would hate it, and it was only once we had driven away that we both discovered that we liked it equally. We arranged further viewings and had the usual searches and surveys done. Though buying the house was not, in some ways, the wisest decision we ever made, we had some happy times there and managed to more than recoup what we had spent on it when we eventually came to sell. In moving, we wanted something like a rural idyll for the children to grow up in, for we had both Rose and Grace by then, and this place was self-contained and secure. The fact that it was miles from anywhere and we would spend the majority of the time that the girls were at school in the car, was not a major consideration at the time, and, if we had thought of it, we may still have gone ahead. Besides, we were cramped in the bungalow. There was a small dining room off the lounge there, separated by an arch through the wall, and I had needed to fit a doorway and double doors to close off this room from the lounge, and had then decorated the dining room as a nursery for Grace, but we felt the need for more space as we were eating off our laps all the time and could not have company over. We definitely had to move to somewhere larger.

The survey on the cottage was not too disheartening, with it highlighting only the need for a new damp-proof treatment to the brick base, and signs of former woodworm and death-watch beetle activity but none were active, allegedly. We had all the exposed timbers treated for both anyway, and some re-plastering was done before we moved in. Almost immediately the central heating boiler broke down, no doubt in protest at having been rudely awoken from its long slumber and put to work. There was also a derelict boiler that had been left on the shingle drive for some time if the pile of desquamated rust on the ground around it was anything to go by, and so perhaps it had not been the best boiler to start with and had just been used as a stop gap until the house was sold. We had the boiler replaced to heat the ancient and flimsy-looking radiators and hoped to retain much of the heat thus produced with the installation of insulation in the roof space, which appeared to have formerly been some kind of recreation centre for starlings. There was straw and nesting material everywhere and multiple breaches in the cracked roofing felt where the birds had gained entry. There was more trouble to come with the roof, though, as the first significant rain that fell showed it to leak like a colander. By going up into the roof with a torch and squeezing past the huge chimney stack that was part of the original building, I was able to identify that every leaded valley in the roof was leaking. A temporary solution was found with the placing of various pots and tubs in strategic places, but we needed a whole new roof before the Winter set in, which was a significant and unexpected expense.

That chimney, apart from being quite a feature, was also shown to work too well. It was open for a fire to be set and had a large copper hood set under it to direct smoke from such a fire upwards and out. When I tapped the hood, apart from appreciating the pleasingly resonant metallic sound that it produced, I was surprised to see some soot drop from it, hover suspended for a second or two, and then shoot up the chimney at a rate of knots. It was good to know that the chimney drew well, but there was simply no point in having central heating when there was also such an efficient method of extracting heat from the house and depositing it into the sky above. Therefore, we had to close off that chimney and so we had a wood-burning stove fitted, which required the addition of a chimney liner, and a supply of wood. Whilst this was a lovely and comforting addition to the room, and we had chosen a burner that looked quite modest for the size of both the house and the room, it soon proved to put out sufficient heat to quickly make the room uncomfortable to be in and drive us from it, so we had to learn how much of a fire we could set to provide sufficient heat to be comfortable but not so much that we could not stay to enjoy it. Once it was going well it also heated up the brick chimney breast which then radiated heat upstairs too. We thought we had got it right after a while, but all that heat seemed to wake up the death-watch beetle which, far from being extinct, had presumably lain dormant in the timber frame waiting for just such an event, and so their tapping became a regular evening accompaniment to our watching of the television. The other thing that was awoken, was a swarm of bees. I went into the lounge one morning to draw the curtains back, only to find the floor carpeted with them, all lined up and ready for action. They were formed into ranks and had each adopted the position of a runner in the starting blocks, with tail ends uppermost and stings protruding at the ready. None of them was flying. I had never come across anything like it before, but I managed to gently remove them, a rank at a time, with use of a soft brush and a dustpan, which I emptied out of the window. None of the bees tried to return and I never knew where they went to having been so rudely evicted from their home in the chimney.

The only other thing about the house that I noticed were the occasional sounds from upstairs which suggested that somebody was walking around up there. This was disconcerting if it happened when all the family and dogs were downstairs, but there was never any feeling of unease or threat within the house, just that comfortable feeling of home. It was only after we had left that Rebekah admitted to me that she had more than once awoken in the night to see the small figure of a boy standing at the foot of our bed, before vanishing. She could not describe him or the type of clothes he wore in the brief glimpse that she had, but she said she felt no fear at those times and sensed only friendliness from him.

I redecorated the place and made it cosy, and we enjoyed being there. After two years of this, Bradley came along to make the family five, and I thought that was enough. Rebekah would have gone on, as her drive to reproduce was clearly strong, miscarriages notwithstanding, but I already felt that a family of five brought its own practical hurdles, such as the size of car needed, booking holidays when most accommodation and travel was based upon two adults and two children, and number of bedrooms needed at home as the girls now had to share, and I did not want more. At least on this I got my own way for once. Fortunately, when I left my first practice, I had more money back from my share than I needed to buy into the next practice, and so we used the surplus to fund another extension to the property. We added two more bedrooms with an adjacent bathroom, a large family room downstairs, with a small entrance lobby and boot room leading from the back door. This gave us much more room for our family and meant it was easier to find some respite from each other if required.

The issue of being in the country brought other considerations too. One thing that I was pleased about, given that we had stabling and paddocks, was that none of the womenfolk in the house wanted to be involved with horses so at least I was spared that expense and worry. If sailing can be likened to tearing up £50 notes whilst standing under a cold shower, then surely owning horses can be likened to a similar destruction of currency whilst being intermittently beaten with a baseball bat or stamped on heavily by a large man in hobnail boots. During my career, I have concluded that some women's association and obsession with horses can only be compared to that of some men and motorcycles. Both are inherently dangerous and liable to cause injury, from the inexperienced riders on entry models, to pushing the boundaries on the higher-octane thoroughbreds, and I have seen parties from both groups with multiple injuries. Even when they get so damaged that they cannot ride, they remain in harm's way, picking up sundry injuries from stabling and grooming on one hand, and mechanical involvement on the other. I suppose the other thing that the two groups have in common is a penchant for waxed cotton clothing manufacturers whose names begin with the letter B. Even now, I live on a road that has a nearby outlet for high-end motorcycles, so that Summer days often attract flocks of people in leather, mostly men, mostly middle-aged, and frequently sporting beards and tattoos. They compare their machines to each other's and lust after those on display and seem equally divided between guys who have ridden all their lives, and those who are new to it, perhaps at some mid-point crisis in their lives which can only be addressed by speed and danger and tight-fitting clothes. These leather-clad desperados also take little practice rides up our road, at considerably greater speeds than the thirty miles per hour limit nominally applied, and accompanied by loud and muscular exhaust output, like a metallic raspberry to all those residents trying to relax and enjoy the weather in their gardens. Fortunately, none of the kids wanted a motorbike either.

We had brought Smidge and Happy, another terrier of the same breed, with us to the new house but we felt that a larger dog might be a good idea and help with security, and so we set about looking for one. This time, we fell on our feet. I was never sure how we ended up looking at the RSPCA rescue centre in Norwich, now long since built upon for housing, but there we were, walking along rows of cages containing hopeful faces. As I walked past one such cage, there came the sound of an object being dropped and then rolling towards us, and a rubber ball came up to the wire frontage, swiftly followed by a moist nose and pair of sad eyes, the owner of which sat down and lifted a paw to the wire. This was Sabre, a German shepherd of unknown vintage, but who was estimated to be possibly two years old. His former owner had left him chained up and alone for long periods and he had developed a habit of licking his forepaws in distress and chewing stones until his teeth were blunted. He and our family took a shine to each other, as we were all present, and times being what they were back then, we soon found ourselves driving home with some paperwork and Sabre sitting in the front passenger foot-well of our car, whining anxiously but not in an unfriendly way. He seemed keen not to spoil this chance that fate had sent him and was the very model of good behaviour. Of course, looking back, I thought we must have been reckless at best, crazy at worst, to have taken him home, but he repaid our trust with interest. Grace was at the stage of bum-shuffling around, having not yet learned to walk, and Sabre would just lie on his bed in the kitchen watching her. Then she developed a habit of sitting between his front and back legs playing, whilst he was laid down on his side but never seemed entirely relaxed, as if he was alert to anything she might suddenly need.

So, I had another dog to walk each morning before work but found Sabre no problem. He slotted right in with the other two and neither side appeared to consider the other a threat. This was quite reassuring to me as I had learned to trust a dog's instincts, and if Smidge and Happy felt that Sabre was OK then I was pleased to take their opinion on it. He was trustworthy and obedient off a lead, and was happy just to lope along, never seeming to tire. I knew that he had some hip dysplasia, a condition that plagues many pedigree breeds, as it had been discovered by x-ray when he was put under anaesthetic to be neutered, but this never caused him any problem. He was also just what the family needed for security for, although he was gentle and trustworthy with us, there was another side to him which was shown only occasionally.

There was an old five-barred gate at the entrance to the property, and we generally kept it open as it was large, heavy, and unwieldy, with an alarming tendency to distort when lifted in order to open or close it. This was fine until an unwelcome visitor entered one day in the shape of the large black male Labrador from the dairy farm half a mile down the road. This dog was never confined and wandered the roads and fields at will. It had never come through the gate before, but decided to this time, and was none too friendly when I tried to persuade it to leave. I did not want an unpredictable dog around where the children were, especially one whose attitude was that he was in charge and had a right to go where he wanted. Sabre obviously detected trouble and wandered over, watched by the confident Labrador who emitted a low growl as Sabre approached. Presumably that was meant as a warning, but it had the opposite effect. In a flash, the Labrador was on its back with Sabre standing over him, with no fight appearing to have taken place. Sabre let the dog up and followed him out of the gate to ensure he had gone and did go to the gate on occasion just to remind any passing Labrador that he was there. However, the Labrador was obviously made of stern stuff and started to approach the property through the large paddock via a gap in the hedge where there was a crossing over the ditch which otherwise surrounded the property. The Labrador was accompanied by a shrewd looking terrier of indeterminate parentage, who was apparently his confederate, and they seemed to mean business. Clearly the Labrador was not happy at being evicted from part of the neighbourhood that it saw as its own and where it had been used to having a free rein. On seeing them in the paddock, I left Sabre at the back of the house and approached them in the longish grass, to be met by another loud warning growl from the Labrador. I decided that discretion was the better part of valour and called Sabre, who came at a gallop, and with a demeanour that clearly said he was delighted to be allowed another go at this interloper and his mate. The Labrador watched him come to within twenty feet, then turned tail and fled, with the terrier bringing up the rear. They never came onto the property again. Because of the outbuildings, there were the cats. That there were vermin around the property was never in doubt. This was never more apparent than during our first Christmas there when the chocolates off the tree kept disappearing and it was found that the resident mice were to blame. They could even be heard scurrying up the tree after the foil-covered booty when we were trying to watch television. Although traps were used in-doors, it was felt that some kind of better deterrent outside would also be good and so cats were decided upon. A charity was found in Norwich which trapped feral cats, neutered them, and then looked for homes for them. This was obviously a challenge as the cats were in no way tamed, let alone house-trained. It was decided that the cottage environment was the ideal place for two of their charges, a ginger and a tabby. Because of their feral nature, and probably because their only contact with humans so far had led to them being surgically separated from a vital part of their anatomy, they were distrustful and shy. They had to have an enclosed area to call their own for two weeks where they would also be fed regularly, after which they could be let out in the expectation that they could still get back to that place for food. A small stable in the middle of the outbuildings was ideally suited and already had a deep layer of straw. The stable door had to be kept shut and I went out twice daily to put down food and water for them, at which points they cowered at the back of the stable, their eyes large and mistrusting. There was no escape attempt at any time. When the two weeks were up, I left the top part of the stable door open for them to decide what to do and crossed my fingers hoping that they liked it there enough to stay. The ginger one left first and went off to make a life of their own, only being seen fleetingly for two or three weeks, and then not at all. No doubt it had gone back to its previous feral lifestyle but without the ability to procreate as enthusiastically as it had previously. The tabby, however, hung around the grounds and seemed to like the new gaff. Part of the ongoing care advised by the charity was to leave food out in the stable so that the cats knew where they could get a meal if they needed. Unfortunately, they seemed not to have kept this to themselves, and so a few new feline acquaintances were formed, of which two were most memorable.

The first was a tabby and white female who started to show up regularly and became reasonably tame. Rebekah went out to the stable one day only to come haring back a minute or two later to say she had something to show me. The "something" was a litter of kittens whose eyes were still closed, and whose fur was still moist at the edges, and who could only have been born the previous night. Clearly the cat had been looking for a safe haven and had been fortunate to find one shortly before her new family arrived. It was decided that the kittens could not be left where they were because of the potential for other visiting cats to harm them, so an old kitchen wall cupboard carcase was brought in from the outbuildings to act as a maternity box and the kittens were brought indoors to the utility room. This took some time for as soon as one kitten had been placed into a cardboard box and another reached for, their mother had retrieved the first one back to the group still reclining in their bed of straw. It took an increase of speed and two pairs of hands before her retrieval was overwhelmed by their removal and the family could be moved en-masse into the utility room. The children, of course, thought they were adorable and spent a lot of time watching and then playing with them. I went in one day to find all the kittens inside the washing machine drum as the door had been left ajar. We felt a certain responsibility towards the mother and her kittens, so decided to arrange for the mother to be neutered, and the kittens to be found homes. By the time we arranged the former, the mother was out and about again, and the vet reported that she was expecting again at the time of the surgery. The kittens were advertised, and all went to good homes for free, though there were many tearful farewells from Rose and Grace on the driveway as they went off with their new families. The girls named the mother Elsa as it seemed she was planning to stay around, and she did just that but always kept her preferred distance from us. If she was seen and we called her, she would trot over for a fuss and a meal but preferred to sort herself out and her hunting certainly helped keep down the rabbit population in the paddock. She was often seen crossing the back garden in the shadow of the hedge, holding a limp form in her mouth, the rabbit not dead but quietened by the hold she had on the scruff of its neck, to be quickly dispatched by a vicious bite to the neck once out of sight and with time to enjoy her meal. The occasional trace of entrails on the lawn were the only other signs of her industry and self-sufficiency. However, Rebekah had wanted to keep one of Elsa's daughters, whom we named Lucky and who was also neutered, but this time whilst *virgo intacta*. She was a much more regular feature around the place than her mother, though still remaining very much an outdoors cat rather than one likely to curl up on the hearth or a lap. The other main character was a male grey cat whom we called George. He was huge, with a thickened and scarred face like a back-street pugilist and a coat that looked like short-dreadlocks until he was cleaned up, to which attentions he suffered uncomplainingly. He seemed to have some blood coming from his back passage, but the vet confirmed that this was due to a hefty load of worms in his bowel, and, once suitably treated, he was in fine fettle. Though we had no knowledge of his provenance, he was clearly a people cat, and loved our company. He ignored the dogs completely and they sort of ignored him too, after realising that all the barking in the world would not cause him to so much as turn a hair, and he clearly was not frightened of them. Perhaps he had experienced and bettered more savage foes than they. He would follow any of the family around like a faithful hound himself, and he loved to be tickled under the chin, at which point he would dribble copiously, which was accentuated by the fact that his canine teeth were slightly longer than normal. He was lovely and nobody in the garden was ever without a companion, though he never tried to come indoors and remained very much his own man. Unfortunately, the lane outside the cottage had become something of a rat-run for cars at peak times and his demise was only a matter of time. I went onto the shed one day and was surprised to see George there but not to have him get up to greet me. Closer inspection showed that this was because he had been run over across the low part of his back and could not move his back legs at all. Quite how he had managed to drag himself off the road and scale the bottom half of the stable door to his one known place of safety I could not imagine, but his outcome was clear. I took him to the vets where he had to be put to sleep. His loss was felt keenly by the whole family, and we considered George to have been an honoured guest who we had been fortunate to have known. The hole he left behind in our lives was never adequately filled.

CHAPTER 14

The garden was my big project. The paddocks were great to have, but I wanted to change the area in which the house sat to something more organised. I viewed the smaller paddock rather as a blank canvas and envisaged making different areas in the garden and encouraging a sense of adventure for the children, whilst keeping it a safe and enclosed space for them to play and explore. The bungalow we had moved from had only a small garden and I had managed the lawn there with a simple push-pull mower, so I had no means to cut so much grass as there was at the new property and just had to let it grow to start with. This had its own attraction as the swathes of long grass rustled and swayed in the summer breezes and did not go on growing beyond a certain length. There was also the constant hum of insects going between the various flowers that bloomed amongst it. Nowadays, wildflower meadows are all the rage for gardening, but I was well ahead of that curve. The second year I managed with a small petrol mower and a scythe for the area that I thought would becoming the garden, but the larger paddock remained doing its own thing.

There were some huge leylandii conifers between our garden and our immediate neighbour in the opposite direction to the dairy farm. These formed a serviceable wind break from the prevailing South-Westerlies, but were unruly, enormous, and their shade darkened the rooms on that side of the house. I knew that this species of conifer could not be cut back hard as they would not sprout new growth from old wood, and so they had to go. Somewhat recklessly, I borrowed a chain saw and associated safety equipment from a patient of mine who was a farmer and I set about the conifers in two stages. I used a ladder to go half-way up each tree and make the first cut and reduce the length of timber that had ultimately to fall, and then got down to the base of the trunk to make a second cut. This way, the length of falling timber was not only shorter but, I hoped, easier to direct. There were practical considerations, of course, like how do you start a chain saw when it needed a foot against it to steady it against the pull on the starter rope. This was clearly impossible up a ladder, but the alternative was to start it whilst on the ground, and then climb the ladder using one hand and with the idling chain saw coughing, grumbling and fidgeting in the other hand. I then had to get to a suitable height, with the ladder appropriately secured, and hold the saw in both hands in order to apply pressure to the trigger to change the idling motor to a roaring beast that threw the chain around the guide bar with a metallic whir, and bit through the tree trunks. All of this was made harder by the need for a hard hat with built in ear defenders and visor, as well as tough leather gauntlets as hand protection. The visor was needed as protection from the stream of dust and debris thrown around by the whirling chain, and the ear defenders as protection from the enormous decibel assault of the motor at full tilt, and much closer to my head than might have been thought wise. I had not been a rural GP for long enough at this stage to have experienced all that could have gone wrong with this arrangement, and I saw plenty of cases later on that showed me how lucky I was not to have injured myself seriously. One such case was an elderly couple who decided to reduce the size of their fire logs by using a chainsaw, but they had no sawhorse. Instead, it was decided that the wife would hold the log steady on the ground with one hand on each end and the husband would operate the saw at the middle of the log's length. All went well until several logs in when the saw bit into a knot in a log and stuck there, which meant that the chain stopped driving the cutting teeth around and through the log, and instead acted like a bicycle chain and propelled the saw forward faster than the husband's reflexes could remove his finger from the trigger and so stop it, meaning it took a rapid jaunt up and over his wife's forearm making a hell of a mess of it. Plastic surgery did a reasonable job of repairing it, but the arm was never quite the same again. Whether it was up to the job of wielding a knife against his testicles one night in revenge, I couldn't say.

After the first tree nearly landed on me whilst I was up the ladder, and only narrowly avoided crushing my foot against the ladder rung, I got the angle of cut and the assessment of wind direction right and the job went well. The only collateral damage was the breaking of one lower spar on the post and rail fence next to the trees from the falling of the top half of that first tree. The kindly farmer who had lent the equipment then brought in machinery to move the cut trees to the bottom of the paddock and then pull up the roots of the conifers and move them to the same place at the bottom of the garden where they lay in rows. After allowing them to dry a bit, I set light to them, where they burned fiercely due to their resin content, and stripped neat lines off the paddock turf. I had taken down the old oak post and rail fencing that had separated the paddock from the gravelled area around the house on two sides and so I used the rails to line the edges of these strips to make identifiable beds that I could use as the vegetable garden. I had to dig all through that topsoil by hand, pulling out roots of weeds and nettles which had managed to secure a good foothold amongst the grass just there. I knew that the nettles were a good sign in a way as they tended to grow best in fertile areas, but they were a terrible tangle to work through. Once the beds were identifiable, I laid weed-suppressant membrane between them and used a wheelbarrow to move load after load of shingle to form pathways between them from a huge mound delivered by tipper truck onto the main driveway. Finally, I surrounded the whole area with wire-mesh fence and a planted a thorny berberis hedge within it to deter rabbits.

For my next project I sourced bare root fruit trees from a nursery north of Norwich and planted an orchard next to the vegetable plot. I took care to mix cooking and eating apples and used some heritage varieties with surprisingly different qualities. There was one with hard, crisp yellowish fruit that had a distinct tang of pineapple when eaten, and another whose white flesh was flushed deep pink once bitten into. I had some pears as well as the apples but decided against trying cherries as I knew that the birds would probably beat me to any fruit unless I netted them, and that was just another thing to do, and could cause injury to any birds who got caught up in the net. I had not accounted for the possibility of deer locally as I had seen no signs, but within a week of planting the trees I found that the bark had been stripped back around many of the trees at a height above the rabbit tubes that I had put on. I kept an eye out and later caught the culprit, a muntjac, in the act as it strolled into the new orchard from the larger paddock and nonchalantly looked around for that morning's snack. It looked most put out when it was chased away from this browser's buffet that it clearly thought had be placed there for its convenience. I therefore increased the height of the protection and added stock netting to the post and rail fences that remained but was not confident of keeping the deer out completely.

I planted a mixed native hedge which completed the separation of the smaller paddock into two areas, with a good area of lawn behind the house, a continuation of that in front and to the side, and the orchard and vegetable plot beyond. This was levelled with surplus topsoil obtained, by that friendly farming patient once again, from digging out the sadly neglected drainage ditches around the property. I reseeded the areas of bare earth or tamed the existing grass where needed, blending the two together. I found this latter task much easier once I could afford a ride-on mower.

All of this left me with a problem. I was now working fulltime, doing nights and weekends on call, running the children all over the place to school and various activities (especially Rose who was nine or ten by this stage) and then I had the garden to tame and maintain. Whilst I enjoyed the challenge and seeing my ideas come to life, this must again have had its effect upon my marriage to Rebekah, despite her having shared this idea to move to the country and live this life. She rarely did anything outside the house. There were signs of disapproval, of course, but I may not have seen them for what they were. When I had fresh produce in the garden, Rebekah would still buy prepared vegetables from the supermarket and take no notice of what was in the garden. If I brought it in to use for a meal then she ignored it, saying she had enough vegetables already. It may just have been that she was showing me that nothing I did was of any value to her at all unless it had been her idea. She never helped with any aspect of what was needed to maintain the grounds but was always quick to point out things that she wanted done. I did not reflect on this at the time, but I was confused by her lack of appreciation of my efforts and lack of involvement in what she had said she wanted to be done. I thought that this was what we had both said that we wanted when we chose to move there, but perhaps the actual practicalities had been forgotten in the romance of the move.

Eventually, several years after we had left the property, the church came back into regular use, and I was invited to a wedding that was held there. It was wonderful to see it brought back to life, and to see the interior with one of those amazing wooden roof structures that are so common in old English churches and see the remaining gravestones well-tended. The occasion gave me a chance for a sneaky peek over the fence to look at what had become of the house and gardens that we had left behind. I was pleased to see that it was more or less as I had left it some dozen years previously, with signs that electricity and water had been brought down to the vegetable plot, and that the short avenue of lime trees that I had planted to lead away from the orchard, and for which I had built a framework to start pleaching them, had grown well. Unfortunately, of the five oak trees that I had planted on the larger paddock to mark the dawn of a new millennium, only one had survived, but that one was doing well and had grown significantly in the interval. I wondered at the time which member of the family it represented.

CHAPTER 15

I enjoyed being a family man but there were many elements to this to be taken into consideration, of which schooling of the children was one such. As mentioned previously, it was Rebekah's wish that they enjoyed a private education, and this meant that Rose started attended a fee-paying school at a tender age, to be followed by her siblings in due course. However, the path did not run smoothly, and I saw a pattern emerge which put me right off the whole idea of private schooling.

All went well at first. Whilst we were at the bungalow near the Broads, Rose went to a Junior School in the northern suburb area of Norwich and loved it and did well. She then moved on to Senior School closer to the city centre and was not so happy. The school was up a hill reached by a narrow and steep drive with no footpath. Some children walked up, and some were driven up to be deposited at the round car park at the top, but the rights of way of the different road users were never clearly differentiated, neither going up nor coming down, so it seemed like every day started and ended with a nightmare. Parents' cars were also lined up waiting along the side of the road for fully half an hour before they need have been, causing general mayhem along there too, affecting through traffic and the passage of buses. Rose did OK there at first, but things seemed to go wrong once she had taken part in a school play. The production was a musical, and Rose had a small part but with a solo song to perform. Although she enjoyed drama, neither Rebekah nor I had particularly noted her singing at home, and it turned out that she had a very good and strong singing voice. She had not been bothered about not being cast in a lead role, but she did want to do the best she could in the part she had been given. However, there was a group number to perform at which point it was clear that her singing voice was better and stronger than that of the lead character, who was also part of that ensemble. I noticed several sharp and meaningful looks aimed by the lead towards Rose, who remained oblivious. There were good reviews for the show, and everything seemed to have passed off well, but then Rose's things started to go missing at school. It was a badminton racquet at first, and it never was found despite a lot of searching apparently being done throughout the school. The next thing to disappear was a hooded navy sports top, and that was where things changed. The pattern that I saw emerge and would see again throughout the children's private schooling time, was that if anyone had an issue, then they became the problem as far as the school was concerned. Rose spent ages searching the school for her top and involved teachers, but to no avail. However, the attitude of the teachers was very much that she had lost it and so had clearly lost her racquet too. The idea that anybody had taken it was simply not considered because "we don't have stealing here". At last, the headmaster became involved and said something about the missing top in assembly, following which it turned up in the music room the same day. Far from deciding that this had been returned by the offender because of pressure from the headmaster, at least one teacher berated Rose for not having looked hard enough, despite Rose having searched the room herself on more than one occasion. Besides, the top had been discovered lying on top of the piano where it would have been very hard to miss by even the most cursory of glances. I felt that this was too much and went to see the headmaster. He tended to take the side of his staff but admitted that there were no other things going missing at the school, to which I suggested that for two things to go from the same person in a short space of time might then imply somebody else being involved, especially if one of the items could be returned once the loss was highlighted as it had been. I also suggested that such a pattern of behaviour from one person to another could be construed as bullying. This produced an immediate response from the headmaster who stated that, of course, there was no bullying at his school, just as he had stated equally vehemently that there was no stealing. I pointed out that whilst denying something was clearly much easier than investigating the problem, it meant that the issue would never be dealt with. The headmaster remained steadfast in his belief that there was nothing that needed to be investigated.

Another issue arose in that I had noticed in Rose's written work that her spelling was not great, but that the spelling mistakes were inconsistent. If a child cannot not spell a word, then they tend to go on making the same mistake consistently. I remember my old English Master at school who always said that the one thing that "Miss" at junior School could be relied upon was to ensure that her charges were unable to spell the word "business" correctly. But then I also remembered this same master being frustrated that so many boys could not spell the word "accommodation" as he said it was so easy to break down into its constituents sounds of ac-com-mod-ation and thus work out the spelling. I had pointed out that it could also be broken down into the more phonetically accurate ac-om-od-ation, to which the master had responded that the word was not spelt that way. I made what I felt to be a reasonable point, which was that the master's strategy to working out the spelling of that, or any, word therefore surely fell down as it relied upon one knowing the correct spelling in the first place. Needless to say, the master did not concede that point and I was probably lucky to avoid a detention for my cheek. But I felt that Rose's pattern of different misspellings pointed to an inability to identify the pattern of letters in a word and might therefore indicate dyslexia. I suggested to the school that she be tested as it would be to her disadvantage if this were overlooked, but they repeatedly declined to do so, saying instead that she was "just slow" and "would pick up" with time and "catch the rest up." They did not actually say "she is just a bit of a dunce" but that was definitely the impression that they were trying to convey to me. We decided to move Rose to a different school based upon our poor experience at that establishment, and also moved Grace, who had done well at the Junior School on the same site. In the meeting with the form teacher on that final term, I was incensed when the form teacher said that she had noticed something about Rose's writing, and had informed the educational psychologist, who had tested Rose and, guess what, had found she had dyslexia! There was absolutely no acknowledgement of my attempts to get them to look into that very matter much earlier, just the beaming self-congratulation that they had uncovered it for themselves and were they not just brilliant at their job? I was pleased the girls were leaving.

The girls moved schools to a different one further out of Norwich, closer to where we now lived and in a dormitory village to the city instead. Rose loved it there as it was smaller and friendly, and she got on well with a little extra input for her dyslexia. Grace, too, got on well there and was clearly of a different nature to her older sister. In time, Bradley also started at the same school in the nursery class, which was co-educational, although the higher school was for girls only. Things were going well until it was Grace's turn to fall foul of the system. Rose had left after GCSEs to do her A levels at a nearby state school, as the cohort size at the private school was too small to support the A levels that she wished to do. The teachers had actively tried to discourage her from her chosen subjects and direct her towards A level courses at the school in which they wanted to boost numbers to make them viable, which should have sounded a warning note that the school was in decline. Grace had never had a problem at either school she had attended and was generally a popular girl in her classes, but then a new girl arrived and seemed to take a dislike to Grace for no apparent reason. One day, I got a call from the school to say there had been an "incident" involving Grace. It transpired that this new girl had come up behind Grace, who was seated at a computer, with an open sheet of paper in her hand, and then pressed it over Grace's nose and mouth and forced her head back into this other girl's midriff making it difficult for Grace to breath, only stopping this because of the intervention of other girls in the class.

On being informed of the details, I made it clear that I considered this to be, not an "incident", but a serious assault, and wanted to know what the headmistress was going to do about it. Of course, following the usual pattern of principals at such establishments in my experience, the answer was nothing, because they did not have a discipline problem or any aggression at that school, and never had done, and Grace had probably done something to incite this response, although they did not know what that might have been. Instead, the headmistress and the drama teacher decided they would do a little cod psychology themselves and, far from separate the girls, which would have seemed the very least response they could have made, they put them together as much as possible, which Grace hated and felt threatened by. The drama teacher also devised a little play that they could both be in. Unbelievably, the teacher wrote the parts so that the other girl's character would smack Grace's character on the bottom "just in play". Grace, of course, absolutely refused to allow this to happen, which was felt by the teacher and headmistress to be just her being difficult and not complying with their efforts to move on from the incident. I was apoplectic at this appalling action on the part of both teacher and headmistress and looked to get Grace out of there as soon as possible. I spoke to the headmistress, but she refused to undermine the actions of her teacher whom, she said, had her full support in this matter, and would not accept that the school had acted inappropriately.

The state school that Rose had gone to for her A levels was very popular and had a long waiting list to join but, fortunately, they made allowances for family members of current pupils. Because she now had a sister there, Grace automatically went to the top of that waiting list and, even more fortunately, a girl in the appropriate year moved house and left, so that a vacancy arose for Grace which we gratefully grabbed. Neither of the girls had any further trouble and loved their new school. I was just left wishing that they had gone to state schools in the first place. It is probably no surprise that the school which Rose had problems at was afterwards subsumed by a neighbouring one, and that which Grace had problems at has since ceased to exist at all.

So that left Bradley, who had shone at the Nursery, but then had to move as the main school was for girls only. He went to the Lower School of a private school in the heart of Norwich and seemed to love it there. There was a blip when the headmaster changed. The previous one also had his wife working there in a pastoral role and they had treated the children there like extended family and were universally loved as a result. The new headmaster seemed much brusquer than the previous one and kept talking about improving the standing of the school through improving the results of the sports teams, and that immediately concerned me. I knew from my own school experience that such priorities rarely advantaged all children equally, and instead they usually encouraged a certain culture within the body of students and parents that was, at best, unhelpful and far from inclusive. Following on from my own experiences with sport, I knew that winning usually meant being encouraged to break as many rules as possible without getting penalised, and I did not think that this was an appropriate thing to encourage in young and developing minds and personalities, however realistic it might subsequently be for the world at large after schooling had finished. The headmaster also got off to a bad start with Bradley, as far as I was concerned, by his actions one Monday morning. Bradley was sitting cross-legged in assembly with the other boys but had a cold and his asthma was troublesome. He had coughed most of the previous night, not slept well, and was tired as a result. So much so, that he could not entirely suppress a yawn during something that the headmaster was saying, which the headmaster took to be an insult aimed at him. He called Bradley out and he had to stay behind and was given a black mark on his record. Bradley never did anything wrong, ever, and had never had a disciplinary mark before, and was devastated. I knew just how he felt, as my son had inherited my own tendency to want to follow the rules. I could not believe that the headmaster could be so self-absorbed that he mistook the action of a tired child as a personal insult, but it told me everything that I needed to know about the new headmaster and likely regime to come. Fortunately, Bradley only had another year to complete, and then he moved to the same state school that the girls had gone to, although only Grace remained there by then. I was pleased that Bradley seemed to have escaped the bullying that the girls had experienced, until talking to him one day about his new school. Bradley said he preferred it as nobody there was clumsy. Asked to explain, Bradley said that in his previous school some of the boys were a bit clumsy and were always knocking into him or treading on his bare feet in the changing room whilst they had their rugby boots on, and other such things. Clearly, the bullying had gone on there too, though at a lower level, and Bradley had not mentioned it so that it could be recognised for what it was. Again, I was grateful for the respite of the state school at which Bradley did very well.

It seemed to me that I had worked myself un-necessarily hard for years just to give the children an experience that I would not have wished upon anyone. I wondered if I were at fault as I did not come from a professional family, and had no background in such schools myself, so my children and us as parents may well have seemed sufficiently different to make them stand out as targets. I simply did not know, but I would certainly not advocate a private education to anyone else. Far from being something to aspire to, it seemed to have been something to avoid at all costs. I realised that some of these petty bureaucracies were badly run and relied upon people not rocking the boat, for they seemed to have no way of dealing with problems. When teachers said, "Are you sure your son/daughter would not be happier somewhere else?" they really meant that they wished that one would move their child so that they did not have to deal with awkward questions or situations. So much easier to ignore issues and blame the victims than to investigate problems properly. This was a pattern that I recognised in other bureaucracies later in life and they normally involved equally self-important but incompetent people.

Another element of family life was the after-school clubs and activities that the children wished to attend or were sometimes forcibly conscripted into. The sheer number, and potential cost of them seemed ridiculous to me, who had got by at school with little beyond the occasional sports fixture and my own ability to keep myself occupied. Rose was the first to be involved, being the eldest, and soon showed a certain ability in racquet sports. She started with tennis, having done well in school and then joining a club outside, and she had some coaching to help her. This, again, was at Rebekah's insistence. Although Rose had a certain talent, and enjoyed the game, she was clearly plateauing in her ability and was not going to be able to take it any further than she had gone. She therefore switched to badminton, and she became good enough to represent the county. This meant she had to attend training after school during the week and go to matches at the weekend. Norfolk was in a group of counties that played each other in a round-robin way, and so there were some long journeys to make for these matches. Somehow, although encouraging the involvement, Rebekah was never involved in these journeys, and I was left to undertake them with Rose and, occasionally, some other team members who needed a lift. I was always welcomed along as the team organisers felt it was helpful to have an unofficial team doctor present. The longest distance to cover was for a match in Nottinghamshire, which was quite some distance to do with a return journey as well as the match to be involved in, but there was also Suffolk, Essex, Cambridgeshire, Lincolnshire and Northamptonshire involved. One of the biggest challenges was the matter of how to help the journey pass as conversation only lasted so long. Initially there was the radio, which was helpful for traffic news, but often boring, especially to Rose whose musical taste varied somewhat from mine. In the end, and because she was mad keen on Harry Potter, I bought the audio tape of Stephen Fry reading the first novel of the series, and we listened to that on journeys. Not only did it last the whole of the longest return journey, but it was able to hold one's attention throughout and help the journey seem to pass more quickly. I was quite happy to listen to the familiar soft vocalisations and characterisation of the novel, but, by the time that Rose felt she had gone as far as she could in badminton, and there were serious exams to study for at weekends instead of training and matches to attend, I did rather know the novel off by heart and was quite happy not to have to hear the dulcet tones of Mr Fry again for a while.

Towards the end of Rose's involvement with badminton she had been joined by Grace, who also showed an aptitude for the sport and who was similarly picked to represent the county. That meant a longer period of taxi service for me, although fortunately Grace was not quite so keen on Harry Potter and preferred her personal stereo and headphones, leaving me to my own music or the radio instead. The evening training, however, was becoming a bit of an ordeal for me, coming, as it did, after a full day's work and being situated at a school sports hall some forty-five minutes' drive away on the other side of the city from where we lived. The training lasted for one and a half hours, but there was no point in driving home only to turn around immediately and come back to collect her. However, one and a half hours was an interminable length of time to have to sit on the low hard school benches, which were the only form of seating for spectators at the training facility. I solved the problem of what to do by going back to the car, which was parked on site, lying down on the back seat, and sleeping the time away. I always seemed to wake up just when I needed to and found it a useful way to retrieve some of the many lost hours of sleep from my nocturnal working.

Grace, however, was not to be distracted by badminton for long, as she had already discovered her major joy, which was dancing. I remember her in the first show that she was in, doing a painfully slow tap routine to the rhythm of the song from Disney's One Hundred and One Dalmatians, *Cruella De Ville*, with a particularly loud stamp on the last syllable. Grace was hooked. The dance school was on the side of the city closest to where we lived, so the driving was less onerous, but more frequent as Grace did classes in ballet, modern, and tap dancing. Various competitions, grades and shows also took time and input, but Grace persevered until she was sixteen. I found myself doing the lion's share of the transport again, unless Grace was involved in a show, at which point Rebekah would insist on going so that she could be seen to be involved and supportive by the other parents.

CHAPTER 16

Bradley was never all that keen on sport and did not push for any after-school activity but was rather coerced into the sports camps that had begun to spring up to fill school holiday time for working parents. These were mostly at Rebekah's insistence as she did not want to have to take time off for child-care during the holidays, and I only had so much annual leave to use. Off Bradley would go, with a sports bag over his shoulder containing kit, packed lunch and a bottle of water, but seemingly with little enthusiasm. I felt a certain sympathy for him and recognised in my son my own ambivalence about such activities. Actually, I would have hated it. Bradley also held firmly to the idea of fair play and found the blatant disregard of it hard to take, especially when the opposite view was also expressed so strongly, and the organisers only really acknowledged the results regardless of how they had been achieved. This even came down to the prizes at the end. The coordinator would call out asking for the winning team of whatever activity it was to raise their hands and would then dispense sweets to them. Of course, some boys would raise their hands when they were not the rightful recipients just to get extra, and no records were apparently made to check, so that the sweets always ran out before some true winners were due to be acknowledged. Fate had dictated that this would normally be when Bradley's team would be called upon, to be met by shrugs and indifference by the coaching staff instead of their rightful reward. Bradley could not reconcile how this could be allowed to happen as it simply was "not fair". Of course, he was correct, but the sweets could be replaced, and I always made sure that I had something in the car for Bradley to compensate for any loss. It was, at least, a gentle introduction to the hard reality of life that he would be having to face and deal with all too quickly and there were echoes of my sports-related incident that showed the casual laziness of authority. The supervisors at the sports camps all had clipboards and pens and could easily have kept a record of the winners and called on them at the end to give out the prizes accurately, but they could not be bothered. There was no negative consequence for the supervisors, they had brought a tub of sweets and handed them out, so job done. They had also not realised that those most likely to miss out were also those least likely to complain about it. In effect, what they were doing was rewarding boys for lying, whilst simultaneously teaching others that rewards for endeavour and success were not guaranteed and could be snatched away from them by others with ill-intent, there was nothing that they could do about it and that those in authority would not care. It may seem only a small matter but this failure to shoulder authority responsibly or to care about the consequences of doing it shoddily is pervasive throughout all levels of society, from sports clubs and schools, through business and work-based bureaucracies, up to local authorities and government departments. The consequences regarding the life lessons that are being taught never seem to be considered. Inevitably there will be some children who toughen up because of these outcomes and become more assertive, but there are others who will withdraw, like a tortoise who peeks out at the world from its shell, sees danger, and so retreats to the only safety it knows, and it is the effect upon these that should be considered for they are likely to fail to reach their potential.

Not all school holiday time was spent in such activity, and we did ensure that they got away once a year on holiday together. We usually went for self-catering apartments or villas, which suited us best in many respects. Firstly, we hired a car for the transfers, which then meant that we were mobile for the duration and could see and do more without the exorbitant extra costs of the trips out organised by the travel company. I always felt that the reps at those initial holiday meet-and-greet receptions on hotel holiday we had initially tried had been keener to sell the excursions than to show anyone where the fire doors were. No commission in fire doors, I suppose.

We always chose decent quality accommodation and were glad to have control over the food we ate. However, once we had made the decision to self-cater and were there in the resort, Rebekah made it quite clear that the family holiday was really *her* holiday, and she did not intend to do anything whilst we were away. I was left with the decision of how much to cook myself, and thus how much food I needed to shop for, and how many meals out I could afford for the five of us. Rebekah, of course, made no contribution to the cost of the holiday or the spending money to be taken with us. Instead, she made large dents in the domestic budget while she prepared for it by buying various toiletries and garments, many of which came back unused.

I found that, for me, the best time of the holiday was first thing in the mornings. I was always an early riser, and being on holiday made no difference, whereas the rest of the family barely stirred before nine o'clock in the morning. Therefore, I could go for a run in the coolest part of the day, enjoying the beach to myself as I ran along the patch of firm sand just above the breaking surf, and then collect some fresh bread and have a fresh coffee before returning to the family and initiating breakfast. One of my loves is good coffee, and I loved being on the continent where you could go into any establishment, however humble, and they would have a proper machine to make proper coffee, unlike similar establishment in the UK at the time whose offerings were much more likely to be suspect. The two were simply not comparable. I relied on a cafetiere at home and then a stove-top moka coffee maker. I had bought a cheap aluminium moka pot coffee maker on one trip away and relied upon that for years, until eventually I was with Suzy, and we got an induction hob in the kitchen and my old reliable would not work on it. Although we also had a well-known brand of coffee pod machine, she could see that I was bereft, and so went out and bought me a moka maker suitable for the new hob, much to my pleasure and gratitude.

When booking a holiday for the family, I always chose accommodation with a barbecue so that I could use this for relatively easy meals of meat or fish, and then accompany them with vegetables or salad, with fruit and ice cream afterwards, so it was not too onerous to be landed with the cooking duties. The time spent whilst one side of the chosen protein content cooked could also be usefully filled by downing a chilled beer, with perhaps a second for the other side or whilst a steak rested. However, especially when Bradley was very young, I had to spend all day keeping an eye on him, keeping him entertained and away from hazards, and attend to changing or toileting needs, whilst Rebekah worked on her tan completely oblivious. Time away was a nice break in sunnier climes for her but was not really a rest for me.

CHAPTER 17

After spending years getting everything just as we had wanted it, I had found the large house and garden more than I was willing to go on managing alone and was mildly surprised to find that Rebekah readily agreed to my suggestion of selling up and downsizing a little. Previously she had expressed the opinion that the size of the house and gardens were what she had a right to expect as the wife of a GP and she had always staunchly resisted my attempts to make such changes before. However, on this occasion she readily agreed and so we arranged valuations and an estate agent was engaged with a view to putting the house on the market for the January. We got through an uneventful Christmas and New Year but, just before the house details were due to be released onto the market, she had turned to me and said,

"When we sell this and I move into my nice new house, I would much prefer it if you were not there!"

No explanation for this had been forthcoming, and the involvement of a third party was strenuously denied.

When it came, the separation of myself and Rebekah was out of a clear blue sky, at least as far as I was concerned. I had been given absolutely no indication that there was anything amiss and, though we were clearly not as close as when we had first got together, I had put this down to the combined pressures of work and home life, and the slipping of our own importance down the league table as the children came along, grew up, and had their own needs and demands. When I thought about it later, of course, the warning signs had been there for some time, but I had remained oblivious to them. I had spent our twenty-year marriage working hard and putting in long hours, including nights and weekends, until only a few years earlier. Rebekah's aspiration was for the children to go to private school, although neither she nor I had experienced private education and the cost of that was an added burden upon my income from the practice where I was a partner. Affording the fees meant that I was forced to supplement my income from the practice by doing extra work for the "out of hours" services. However, I could not argue with the fact that my work commitments, of all sorts and for whatever reasons, had kept me from home more than I would have liked. Also, despite all the school runs that I did, as well as my stints doing the family taxi services running the children to various after-school and holiday clubs and activities, Rebekah clearly believed that by working as much as I did, despite her reaping the financial rewards of this, I must have shirked my responsibilities at home.

There was one point in our marriage where I can see that our paths were diverging now that I look back. I have never really liked music gigs, except at a venue where everybody remained seated. Two that I particularly remember were to see Elton John at Carrow Road football ground, and George Michael at Wembley Arena. However, after this second gig Rebekah did say that she would have enjoyed it more with somebody else as I was not much fun. This is not really what you want to hear from your wife. Rebekah loved a more frenzied crush at a music event, and so increasingly she went looking for that environment. She and a girlfriend would drive for hours across the country to some arena to see Michael Jackson or Robbie Williams, endure a long queue to park the car, and then several hours of standing around waiting for the venue to fill up and night to fall before the stage came alive for a couple of hours. She would then wait for a further couple of hours to get out of the car park before the long drive home again. I could never see the point in that as the couple of hours of entertainment in no way compensated for almost a day of inconvenience and discomfort. Perhaps it was then that she decided that her future was not going to be with me and so started to look in a different direction.

I had also been improving and maintaining our period home and three acres of grounds, which was similarly viewed by her as "time off" from being a father and husband. Looking back, I remembered that there had been the appearance of a mail order, battery operated, hand-held leporine device of hers, secreted within her wardrobe and which I had stumbled across whilst I was in search of paperwork for a holiday. I also remembered that the box it was in showed signs of having been opened a sizeable number of times. As well as this, Rebekah had been going on increasing numbers of evenings out with "new friends" whom she had apparently met through work but who never came to the house. Although I had barely noticed it at the time, I could clearly recollect the time she had come home from her part-time nursing job and enthused about a "lovely bloke" that she had met that day, a patient that she had attended to but whose chief distinguishing characteristics seemed to be that he lived alone after a clean-break divorce, drove a Porsche, and had no children of his own. In due course, I was told that an invitation had been extended to her by this man, one Colin Gudgeon, to go for a ride in the Porsche as she had never been in a sports car before. I consented but did not really feel that my permission had been sought and I was sure that she would have gone regardless of my reply. I did, however, remember vividly that she had driven a sports car in a session around the Lotus factory test track as I had bought that experience for her as a birthday present the previous year, and she had enjoyed it immensely, so she certainly was not without sports car experience. At least, not of the driving sort. I wondered if perhaps there was something fishier to this man that just his name, especially as the trip in the Porsche had eventually taken all day and had included her being treated to lunch, but when questioned she vehemently denied that there was anything more to it. Of course, long after the separation she eventually admitted that there was more to it, and Rebekah and Colin subsequently married. It might have been love at first sight between them, but then he was single after a clean-break divorce with no children to complicate the picture, living in his own house with just a few years left on the mortgage, driving a flash car and having a millionaire father. Perhaps all that was just coincidence. I personally don't believe in coincidence but do believe that if the same guy had been penniless, living in rented accommodation, paying spousal maintenance and with a few kids in tow to manage then she wouldn't have looked at him twice, let alone allowed him into her knickers. She resembled nothing so much as a monkey making its way through the treetops, never letting go of one means of support until she had a good firm grip on the next and holding onto both for as long as was possible.

On our last family holiday abroad the summer, before the separation but after the spin in the Porsche, we had a three bedroomed apartment After sharing a bed with me on the first night, Rebekah had declared it too uncomfortable and had moved out. She had then spent every night of the remaining time away either sharing with one of the girls or sleeping on a sofa, both of which she declared preferable for comfort to the double bed that we had shared on that first night. I had been perplexed but compliant, though I could not really understand her behaviour. Now, of course, all had become clear. I don't know why the penny had not dropped sooner, but as Suzy would later point out to me intelligence and common sense were two flowers that rarely bloom in the same garden, and they certainly did not seem to in mine.

In later years I had time to reflect upon the impact that a molar pregnancy and several miscarriages may have had upon our marriage and whether they had started to lead Rebekah down a different path. The molar pregnancy was her second, after Rose, and she had attended the dating scan on her own as work commitments meant that I just could not get away. When she phoned to say that they had found something that was not a baby, she sounded so scared and bewildered, having expected a happy event but having been given grave news instead. In a molar pregnancy the placental cells proliferate and overwhelm the foetus so there is no baby, just an invasive and dominant placenta that looks like a bunch of grapes on an ultrasound scan. She needed a procedure to remove this from her womb, and weeks of tests to ensure that levels of the placenta marker, HCG, had dropped to normal because a rise could indicate that some tissue had been missed whereupon it can act like a cancer and invade the womb lining. It can also be resurrected by future pregnancies, so the condition cast a cloud over each successive pregnancy as well. The fact that several of these ended in miscarriage added further jeopardy. The cause for the miscarriages was eventually discovered to be Systemic Lupus, a condition where the body produces antibodies against its own DNA. When our last child, Bradley, had been successfully delivered, the midwife commented about how we had suffered for our family, but there is no doubt that Rebekah suffered more than I did. Perhaps that is why she felt the children were so precious to her that she could not bear to share them with me after our divorce. If that was the case then she clearly had never considered that I had also suffered hurt and loss, and a sense of helplessness. Although we were both upset after each loss, we never really discussed the impact upon us either as individuals or as a couple, and it may have been that Rebekah felt let down by me because of her obstetric difficulties despite my medical knowledge. Or perhaps the losses left her with an insecurity that was not helped by my work-related absences from the home. If that was the case, however, she never let me know this even when she wanted the separation. Whatever her issues with me were, she had clearly found something or someone that she thought was better and felt there was no point in discussing her reasons as they would make no difference in the end. The fact that she had chosen an alternative without ever pointing out what was the problem in the first place was hurtful, however, and her subsequent actions merely seemed vindictive and manipulative.

However, despite the surprise and shock, I found myself making the entire process much easier for Rebekah than she had any right to expect. When the split with Rebekah came, I was far too accommodating. I allowed the situation to be explained to the children as if it had been a mutual decision, and one that had been arrived at after significant consideration and discussion, rather than the unilateral diktat that had actually occurred. I did not know why I did that, but I presumed that somehow I was trying to soften the blow for them, and I did not want there to be any apparent antagonism that might affect their future relationship with either of us. I knew that the least damage was inflicted on the children by a separating couple if they could remain in touch and on good terms with both parents, and I did not want to start apportioning blame or indicating that the children should take sides. After all, who was to blame? Rebekah may have said the words, but was that really such a shock, or so far from what I had thought myself? I no longer felt attracted to her, and had not done so for some time, and it could be argued that, in my mind at least, it was me who had first left the marriage. I had been there in body, of course, doing all the things I had ever done to keep the family functioning and household running, but my heart was not really in it, and I did it out of a sense of loyalty and for the family as a whole rather than for her. Sex had become something done out of duty rather than desire, perfunctory and performed without enthusiasm, rather like the kiss from a child on the whiskered face of an aged great aunt. It cannot have been doing anything for Rebekah either, if that device in the wardrobe was anything to go by. Of course, children are not stupid and may have picked up on this undercurrent themselves. Perhaps the confirmation from us both about the separation was actually just a culmination of what the children had suspected and feared for some time – I never found out either way.

So, I sorted the finances, arranged for the house to be sold, which went through very quickly, and looked for the next step for us all. I found a nice four-bedroomed detached house for Rebekah and the children, close to her work as a practice nurse, and to the children's school, and that she was happy with. I also found a smaller three bedroomed one for myself which was near enough to my practice to nip home at lunchtime to see to the dog who was to come with me. At this point I still believed the lie that Rebekah had told me which was that the separation was just a trial for six months or so, and so I had an eye on the future use of this smaller house as a rental if we reconciled and I moved back with the family into the larger one. Although my feelings for Rebekah were gone, I had no intention of looking for anyone else and would have been content enough to see things through until the children left home. I did not know about the presence of Colin until several months later, when I had finished all the renovating that Rebekah wanted done on her property. I stripped and refitted wardrobes, scraped off peeling emulsion from ceilings and coving where the surfaces had not been sealed, applied diluted PVA to remedy the situation, and repainted them with several coats of white emulsion. I fitted out her airing cupboard with shelves which had to be removable to allow access to the central heating boiler which was situated at the back of the cupboard. I put lighting in the loft as well as a run of tongue-and-groove flooring up there and decorated anywhere else in the house that needed it, be it in a bedroom, bathroom or kitchen. Only then, when all of the tasks were completed, did I find out that there was somebody else in her life who could have done all of that, but, of course, she had let me do it for her and at my own expense. And suddenly, once I knew the reality of the situation, I became persona non grata at that address except for when I came to collect the children for the school run every morning. Even then, I had to wait at the curb or in the car and was not allowed to come to the door. Also, I was driving well out of my way to take them to the school that was just up the road from their mother's house, and then drive back in the other direction to go to work myself. Was there no limit to my stupidity? Apparently not, but I did it out of a sense of determination to keep the children's lives as consistent as possible.

Well, at least I got the divorce in motion. Whilst all was well, before I found out about Colin, we had approached a mediator and gone through all the finances and come to an agreement. At that point we had to take it to our own solicitors to settle this in law, and that was when the trouble started. The immediate response of Rebekah's solicitor was that I was trying to get her out of her house. Although I was not, and nothing could have been further from the truth, Rebekah's attitude immediately changed, and she became combative. My view was that this was a deliberate tactic by the solicitor to stir up trouble and argument as there was more money to be made out of acrimony than agreement, and that certainly proved to be the case.

Initially, I was prepared to allow Rebekah to divorce me, but, somewhat belatedly, reality kicked in. I realised that I could not see what I had done wrong, and that being the "guilty" party might make the children believe that I had done something that they were not aware of. Therefore, I insisted that I divorce Rebekah and fortunately, though the causes I cited were not agreed by her, neither were they contested.

The divorce followed its stumbling progress, and the decree absolute came through, but somehow, I never got my copy. The children were still coming over to my house at the weekends at that point, and subsequently I wondered whether the decree had arrived on the mat whilst they were staying there, and one of them had taken it. It would be just like their mother to ask them to look out for solicitor's letters to copy, or photograph on their phones, or simply just take. And it would be just like them, I reflected, to comply with that instruction. They had started off seemingly pleased to come over and see me, but gradually they had come for less time, and been in almost constant text contact with their mother whilst at my houses. Rose came in her car but only on the Sunday afternoon and she took Grace home with her whilst Bradley stayed so that I could take him to school the following day. Grace turned up by bus at six or seven o'clock in the evening on a Saturday, usually keeping everyone waiting for the evening meal, then went to her bedroom early. She then got up around mid-day on the Sunday, just in time for a lunch before then going back with Rose. I did not really see how the word "access" could be used to define my relationship with my middle child under those circumstances. Eventually Grace stopped staying altogether and just came with her sister for a meal on the Sunday. She was keen to dictate events, including by her diet. She had been vegetarian for a few years but became vegan during this time. Her views had not changed radically and so it seemed that this was merely a way of trying to exert control over part of her life whilst other parts were beyond her doing so. I felt that, if anything, I preferred that she tried to control the content of her food rather than the quantity of it and would rather that she followed a discipline such as veganism than develop a more formal eating disorder that could adversely affect both her physical and mental health.

I tried to be accommodating in this. I baked vegan buns and prepared vegan food for Grace. There was always too much for her to get through over the course of the weekend, and I offered the surplus to her to take back home. However, Grace was not allowed to take it back with her. She had made it clear that nothing from my house was allowed to "contaminate" her mother's home or existence. At this point Grace was better inclined towards me and had even asked if she could move in with me as she said that she was not getting on with her mother at that time, although she did not go into details about why that was. I did not dismiss the idea but wanted her to know that I thought she should continue a good relationship with both parents and asked if there was any particular thing I could help with. She said not, went back to her mother's as usual, and all went quiet again, until the following Spring.

CHAPTER 18

She had been there, under my nose all the time, but I had simply not noticed her. Suzy mentioned later that she was not surprised, really. I had built my defences so high, and so impenetrable were they, that I could probably not look out on the world at all. Suzy had joined the practice as a receptionist, with many years of reception work experience in the NHS behind her. I had barely noticed the new face. I was not unpleasant, I was never unpleasant to anybody, but I did not engage and was just brusque and business-like. I was aware that she was with somebody as that man had accompanied her to the Surgery's Christmas party, but that was all. Suzy later told me what a sad and lonely figure I had cut at that same party. I was still with Rebekah, and it was before her statement regarding the house move, but she had cried off attending the function and I, as partner, had a responsibility to be there. I sat alone, chatting where needed, but mostly keeping to myself. Suzy said that her heart went out to me, but there was no instant attraction, and she never had any thoughts that we might end up together. Indeed, she said that she had thought me increasingly aloof and stuck up at work, so uncommunicative was I. In fact, her exact phrase was that I acted as if I had a pole stuck up my arse. She later realised that I was hurt and had essentially built some high and robust defences against it happening again, such that nobody could get in. On hearing this, I subsequently wondered whether that had unwittingly contributed to my children's subsequent defection – had I built them so high and thick that they had failed to penetrate too? If that were the case, though, why did their defection not occur until after I had started a relationship with Suzy, as surely those defences must have been breached a little by that event.

The change, when it came, came slowly, like the gentle thawing of a frost in the late Winter sunshine. The practice had a little branch surgery in a village a few miles away from the main one. The building was owned by the parish council, but it accepted a nominal rent (I seem to remember it was a single rose on the First of May, though whether any roses actually changed hands I did not know) in exchange for the practice holding surgeries there as a benefit to the inhabitants of the village and its immediate environs. When I had joined the practice there were three such surgeries held each week, but this had subsequently dropped to two mornings per week. Within a few years even these stopped, and the branch surgery closed. Audit undertaken by the practice had showed that most patients seen at the branch surgery had travelled there from elsewhere in the practice merely because that was where the next available appointment was, and that most patients from the village where the branch surgery was situated had actually travelled to the main surgery to be seen. Certainly, the branch surgery had the doctor and the receptionist, but only basic equipment, and no nurse input. Anything that was not simple had to go to the main surgery to be followed up anyway, so it was not an efficient use of the doctor's time. The death knell for the branch surgery came when the Care Quality Commission inspected the premises and deemed them unfit for purpose as they were too small and had no confidential space at reception as this was merely an open desk in the middle of the small waiting room. The consulting room door also opened onto that room, and I could hear patients talking in the waiting room even with the door shut, so presumably there must have been a fair amount of verbal traffic audible the other way around too. Also, there was no access or specific toilet facilities for disabled patients, and the ceiling covering of polystyrene tiles was a fire hazard. The practice could not make changes as we did not own the building and would not have done so if we could as the building would have had to have been razed and then rebuilt, and it was simply not worth it to do that. There was some resistance to the closure, mostly amongst residents of the village who were not patients or who had not attended the surgery for some years, but who wanted to be seen to be politically active amongst the community, presumably with some other ambition in mind. Once we had abandoned the building to the parish council's auspices again, it became a fish and chip shop. I hope they changed the ceiling tiles first.

Be that as it may, at the time I did the regular Thursday morning surgery there. I was accompanied by one of the long-serving receptionists, and it was usual practice for the doctor to drive the receptionist there, as parking space was at a premium, and then drive her back to the main surgery afterwards, by way of any home visits that had to be done. After Suzy had been in post for nearly a year, the receptionist who normally accompanied me left, and the Practice Manager chose Suzy to go in her place. So, Suzy and I, forced together into my car by circumstance, got chatting in a way that we would otherwise never have done. We found that we had much in common. Suzy loved to cook and bake. Indeed, she often brought in trays of cakes that she had made for the staff and those brownies and flapjacks had brightened many of my morning coffees over the preceding year. I, too, had always cooked to a certain level, having started when a student at university, and was, by then, living alone and managing for myself and the children when they were over. We each brought in examples to share on a Thursday morning, and I found that the coffee I was being brought in the consulting room was suddenly of a higher quality than I had come to expect from the jar of instant that normally supplied the branch surgery and from which a spoonful of granules had to be chipped from the caked accumulation in the bottom. And then there was our shared love of dogs. I had Mully the dalmatian whose name was another nod to Peter Cook and referred to The Ballad of Spotty Muldoon. Suzy had Bibby who was an almost snow-white golden retriever. Although purchased at Rebekah's insistence following the loss of Sabre, Mully had always been my dog really, and I had kept him during the separation, being fortunate that I was able to divert from home visits to my new home to let him out at lunchtimes on a workday. One glorious summer day, just as we were pulling away from a home visit, I mentioned that it would be lovely if we did not have to return to work on such a day but could go and walk our dogs instead. I had not intended this to be together, but that was the way that Suzy understood it and she agreed. She had separated from her partner by that stage and was living in rented accommodation with her daughter and Bibby. Of course, the working day progressed as normal for us both, but the incident had planted a seed in my mind. I had not been looking for anyone, but company would be nice and so, that following weekend, with the weather still lovely, I phoned her to see if we could take that walk together. Unfortunately, she was busy shopping with her mother, but, before the call ended, she expressed the hope that I would offer again. I did so, on the next weekend that I did not have the children to stay, and we agreed to meet up. Suzy gave me her address and I duly arrived with Mully in the back of my estate car. I met Bibby, who seemed a little haughty about a canine intruder into her domain, and I caught a brief glimpse of Mary, Suzy's daughter. We loaded up, took the leads and fresh water for the dogs, and drove to the coast, to walk along a shingle beach with the sun shining, a fresh breeze blowing, and the surf sparkling. The dogs got on well enough, and we both found that we could talk easily to one another. By the time we turned around at the end of the stretch of beach and walked back, I was wondering whether it would not be a good idea to hold her hand. She offered no objection to this and by the time we had got back to the car park, a kiss seemed the most natural thing in the world. Without ever really meaning to we had started a new chapter together.

There followed further walks, and we took turns to host each other for dinner, occasionally staying over, each bringing our dog at the same time. The relationship grew and developed quickly. I met Mary soon after and we got on tolerably well. Time was to see this improve, but there was no real issue at the start. I could see how she could manipulate her mother with promises she did not intend to keep, and downright lies at times, but I soon learned not to point these out to Suzy, as her immediate reaction was to leap to her daughter's defence. Mary's father had been an older man and had passed away a few years earlier, so the potential for awkwardness there was avoided and, eventually, I assumed the role of father figure in her life. But that was still in the future at this stage.

My own children, however, were not so accommodating. They were pleasant enough in their manner, but their resistance showed. Initially I did not see Suzy on the weekends that I had them to stay with me, but there was no reason for this to be a prolonged arrangement. After all, their mother had introduced Colin to them within two weeks of our separation without any problem so there was no reason to presume they needed protection from how my life was changing, and there was no reason to let them think that they had the power to control what I did or who I saw in my own life. However, the potential problems were apparent on the first day that they were there, and Suzy came over. She walked into my lounge where the children were sprawled watching TV, and none of them even acknowledged her presence, let alone moved to allow her to sit. She chose not to bring this to my attention, as I was in the kitchen cooking Sunday lunch for us all, but it was definitely a sign of things to come. It might have been that the children looked to me for a bit of stability in their lives whilst her mother settled into the new relationship that she had broken up the marriage for. Similarly, it may have been that I had disappointed them a little by not remaining always available to them and with no call on my time other than them or it may just have been that Rebekah chose to exert the influence over them that she most definitely had. Be that as it may, there was no reason why I should not have been allowed to move on with my life in the same way that Rebekah had so clearly done, and I was determined to do so.

The crunch came some six months after the relationship between Suzy and I had started. It was in the middle of a freezing spell of January weather, and the boiler in Suzy's rented house broke down leaving her without heating or hot water. The landlord was equally glacial in his speed of response and so, after two weeks of this, I decided it would be best for Suzy and Mary, together with Bibby, to move in with me. I had the room for them, and the house was warm. This arrangement worked well, but there was a need for Grace to share a twin room with Mary when she came over. I reasoned that this was only one night a fortnight so she would just have to manage it, but Grace clearly thought that this was a step too far. She stopped staying over, although did come over with Rose on alternate weeks. However, one day in April, she stated that she did not want to come over at all, and, in fact, did not want any further communication with me. She said that her mother had "told her everything" and that she wanted to stop all communication as a result. She would not contact me, did not want me to contact her, and would inform me if this situation changed. I asked, reasonably enough I thought, what the "everything" was, and would she not like to hear my version. In reply she said that she believed what her mother had told her, though still did not say what this was, so if I said the same as her there was no point, and if what I had to say was any different then I would be lying, and she was not about to sit and listen to any of my lies. I was shocked. I knew that I had done nothing to the children to account for this stance of theirs, for Rose subsequently joined in on her sister's side, and I could not account for the unfairness of the position that they had adopted. But there was little I could do against their fierce determination to keep me out of their lives. They were in their middle and late teens and so of an age where they presumably knew their own mind, and I just felt that they would reconsider in time. Rose did eventually do just that, although it took nine years, but Grace still stayed aloof and out of touch. I sent text messages on their birthdays and at Christmas, as I did not feel that a card would get past their mother's censorship at the front door, but they did not reply. So why the turnaround from Grace? Had the idea of moving in with me been a test or was there really a problem at her mother's house that required Rebekah to act and "tell her everything". Who knows? Certainly not me, who still did not know why she had asked to move in with me in the first place, or why she then made the decision that she would not come in future. It did make me remember an earlier comment of Rebekah's though, where she had said that I had no interest in my own children, now that I had a new "daughter", Mary. This was not true, of course, and I had just thought her ridiculous at the time, but perhaps this was what she had been telling the girls, and when Suzy and Mary moved in with me, they had seen this action as confirming what their mother had been saying to them all along. Whatever the case, their separation from me was absolute. They ignored all my attempts at communication with them, despite me persisting with this for several years.

Although we could manage in my three-bedroomed house, Suzy and I realised that we needed more room, now that there were three of us and two large dogs, and so we started to look for something a little larger. We were fortunate to find a newly built four-bedroomed house not far away, with good-sized rooms and space to stretch out a bit. The garden was larger for the dogs too, and there was a park and countryside walks on our doorstep. We were also closer to the city and all of its services. There were all sorts of dark rumblings from Rebekah about how things were moving a bit too quickly to last, and how I was probably "Thinking with my cock and not my head". She always did have an elegant turn of phrase. However, both Suzy and I felt certain we were doing the right thing.

CHAPTER 19

Once we had moved to the larger house, things seemed on a more even keel. Bradley was coming over regularly and had his own room which was of a better size than the box room he was used to at my previous house. He seemed to be more settled, and things followed a regular pattern. He was going through adolescence, with its hormonal upheaval and attendant social difficulties, and he seemed to be very comfortable discussing with Suzy all of the confusion and uncertainty he was going through. Although she only had a daughter, Suzy was empathetic to his woes and worries and helped him enormously with good advice and encouragement. He would arrive from his mother's house clad in woeful garb for a teenager, with ill-fitting jeans, bulky Velcro-strapped trainers, and baggy t-shirts, the latter being bought deliberately several sizes too large by his mother to allow ample room to grow. Suzy and I took him into the city to get some better fitting, and more befitting, clothes so that he would not stand out from his peers when meeting them at weekends and in the holidays, and thus aggravate his already obvious social awkwardness. He liked these and took to them easily, but over time we noticed that that he started to come over from his mother similarly dressed. He was never allowed to take the new clothes that I bought him to her house, in the same way that Grace had not been allowed to take food back in the past. Indeed, he would quake at the suggestion that he might do that, but Rebekah had no compunction about sending Bradley to mine in those clothes that she had bought him. They were not allowed to be washed at our house and he had been told by his mother that he was no longer allowed to wear the clothes that I had got him whilst over with us either, apparently because otherwise the clothes that his mother had bought him would not get enough wear to justify their cost. I could only marvel at the level of control that she obviously craved and enjoyed, even at a distance. She clearly just got off on it.

But it was not just the clothes where Suzy helped. Bradley talked to her about his confusion over girls and any crush that he had, as he really did not know what to do. There were bodily changes too, and emotional confusion, all of which Suzy listened to and talked about with patience and insight. I could certainly identify with that part of growing up and was not sure that I could have offered any practical or meaningful advice so was grateful for Suzy's listening ear and helpful input. Bradley never really approached me about any of that. I had similarly never talked to my father about such matters but with my knowledge and medical experience I at least felt equipped to help Bradley out, despite his preference for Suzy. Fortunately, she shared the conversations with me and made it clear to Bradley that she would do, unless he specifically asked her not to, which was rare. I also helped develop Bradley's independence. I realised that his mother and sisters might censor any written communication with me, so I bought him his first mobile phone so that we could keep in touch, as Bradley did not have one at that point and his mother apparently disapproved. Of course, this may have been a lie as she certainly made good use of it, once Bradley had it, both to keep track on him and to send her orders to him, and there was never any chance that he would have tried to conceal its presence from her as he was too much in her thrall. That was one item from my house that he was encouraged to take to hers.

Another of the things that I had done to help with his independence was to take Bradley onto the buses locally and into Norwich, as his mother did not want him to use them. This was frustrating for Bradley as he was also thirteen by then and in need of some independence and socialising at weekends. Therefore, I took him on the bus up to Norwich, showing him what to ask for, where the bus dropped him, and where the return bus stop was to get home. However, having initially opposing Bradley's new-found independence, Rebekah embraced it wholeheartedly when she realised that it meant that he could get the bus to school, so this is what was done. This had the added bonus to her that I need not come anywhere near her house in order to collect Bradley for the school run. It also meant that there was no need for her to do anything more than pack him off on the quarter mile walk to the Market Cross at the town centre to pick the school bus up. Therefore, I stopped taking Bradley to school every day, but I did pick him up on a Wednesday evening after school, where upon he stayed overnight with us, and I then drove him back to school the following day. When it was my weekend to have Bradley to stay, Bradley came on the bus, and stayed until the Monday morning school run, again done by me. This seemed to be no problem at all to Bradley. At our house he had a large room to himself. Indeed, it was much the same size as his room at Rebekah's house, and he had a desk and laptop to do his homework on. However, if there was anything new in the house, he noticed it immediately and would comment upon it. Many of these comments related to the potential monetary value of the item, hence my view that he was taking notes to report back to Rebekah. It was as if he acted as his mother's eye and ears in my house and he did not miss a trick. When my father died, Bradley even had the nerve to ask what I had been left in his will, no doubt to report back to his mother for her to attempt to get a share. Fortunately, I could be quite truthful and say that I had received nothing as everything had rightly gone to my mother, but it just showed me what a long way they had come from the children that I thought I had known.

Bradley did start to make several comments that indicated that perhaps his mother and sisters were not altogether pleased that he was still coming over, but it was still a great surprise that he suddenly stopped coming. There had been no prelude, but he announced one Sunday evening in January, three years after the girls had taken their leave, that he intended to do the same. There had been no warning, no intimation of any problem, just the resolute statement on the Sunday evening that this would be the last time that he would come to my home, or even contact me, for the foreseeable future. There was some mention of "seeing how things were after a few months", but I had heard that one before and now knew what it really meant. That is your lot, sunshine. The timing was significant as well. Grace was just about to turn eighteen, and child maintenance would no longer be payable for her by me to her mother. As Bradley would no longer be staying with me, the maintenance that I had to pay for him would rise, and the increased amount just about covered the shortfall that Rebekah would otherwise have had to endure. Could a mother be that mercenary about her own children that she would seek to manipulate their contact with their father purely for financial gain? Well, I had no doubt that Rebekah could, and was doing so.

I tried the text messages on birthday and Christmas as I was still doing to the girls, but, after a further year of no replies from any of them, I called it quits and stopped any attempt at all. Bradley seemed to have been welcomed back fully into the fold at his mother's after fraternising for so long with the enemy, and Facebook was full of happy family shots of them all together and with their new extended family.

I found a bit about their lives from Twitter and any other on-line presence I could access but I had to be content with those crumbs about their life and how they were doing, until a text from Rose after nine years of nothing.

So how did the absence from my life of anything to do with my children actually feel? I felt as if a large part of my life had been suddenly ripped away and I struggled to reconcile what had happened with any kind of justification. I had been offered none, and I presumed that Rebekah and the children felt that none was warranted, but it was just one of the things which kept me awake at night for months and years afterwards. I simply had no idea what was it that I was meant to have done or said that would have made such a difference. The hardest part was trying to shut off my imagination. I could think through any number of future scenarios when I might reasonably have been expected to be involved in their lives but was now unlikely to be. When sleep failed to come in the wee small hours, I would run these over in my mind again and again, never managing to come to any conclusion, and gaining no comfort from the lack of outcome. I thought about Bradley finishing school – what would he do, and where would he go? What were his aptitudes and ambitions? I no longer knew. I had no idea what Grace might do, and this was made more difficult by her failing to get reasonable grades in her A levels, causing her to have to re-sit them. This meant that she missed that year's university intake, and actually then never did go. Later, I found out that she worked in insurance and was vaguely aware that she was in a relationship and had then moved in with her partner, but I was woefully short of details.

Then there was Rose – I knew that she had gone to university and was able to follow her progress there. But for each of them, it was the potential future that I could not help thinking about. What were they to do, and where? Where would they live and with whom? Would I ever see them married, and what about grandchildren? I knew of families where the grandparents never got to see their own child's offspring and they never stopped thinking about what might have been. It is almost impossible to quantify the misery that one's own thought processes can inflict in the absence of any specific knowledge or hope. It was also difficult to establish who was to blame. I immediately thought it was Rebekah, of course, and her attempt to command as much of my income as possible, as well as control as much as possible. But was that it? Were our children so easily convinced, or was this their own idea? If so, then what had caused it? If they were so content to let their mother move on after the marriage, then why not allow me the same outcome? Or was it more than that - had I actually done something to hurt them, or keep them at a distance from me? Then back to those night-time ruminations, looking for what I might have done. I reflected upon all the things that had passed, what my motives had been and how they might have been interpreted, but I could not come up with any concrete answers.

In the end, the passage of time just seemed to take the edge off my anxiety about it. It never went away, and occasionally

I picked at the scab that formed over the wound, sometimes just to see if it still hurt. I was not sure if a time would come when it no longer did and, if that happened, then what I would think about that situation. Would that be a relief from this endless soul-searching and insomnia, or a sadness that I had become numb to the hurt? Would I feel that I had somehow let my children down if their loss from my life was no longer as raw as it had been? However, I also had to think that, if I had done something, then my children were complicit in this loss by not informing me of the perceived slight and allowing me to explain. They were clearly at least content with the status quo.

Eventually, after several years, I found that thoughts of the children drifted from the forefront of my mind. They were still there, easily within reach if required, but needed less and less. There were only so many times you could get on the merry-go-round of self-inflicted pain with no outcome, before the idea of the ride became off-putting. I thought of them, of course, if something came up to remind me of them, or a song on the radio, a book on the shelf, a subject on the television that I thought that one of them would have liked, and, of course, there were always the birthdays and other significant events through the year. I became a spectator of Father's Day after my own father had passed away, having no contact from my own children. I also felt for my parents and their loss of the children too. It was amazing how many families that I knew of where the grandparents had become peripheral figures, if they figured at all. I remembered having respect for my grandparents but found that this seemed increasingly rare in society around me. I reflected that what I felt was not unlike a bereavement with regards to the initial shock, hurt and anger that I had felt, followed by the ceaseless attempts to process why and how, only to eventually move to a point of a grudging acceptance of the situation without forgetting them or some of the happier times we had shared. I did, at least, have the potential of reconciliation with those lost to me, however remote that possibility was. It was a chance that many others, bereaved by death, did not have, and I was grateful for that at least.

CHAPTER 20

Throughout all of this time I had a relationship to develop with Suzy's daughter Mary, who was to become my stepdaughter, and this proved a challenge. The main problem for me was that I was never really sure of just where I stood in this regard. Suzy had her challenges with Mary but seemed somewhat ambivalent about what she wanted. She might espouse all sorts of frustrations about Mary and her behaviour, but if I were to agree with her or mention these issues myself, Suzy would immediately jump to Mary's defence against me. As a colleague mentioned to me at the time, if there was one thing worse than having a seventeen-year-old in the house, it was having somebody else's seventeen-year-old there.

The first thing that I found was that Mary seemed sullen. Suzy was determined that this was just a natural shyness, but I thought otherwise, especially as she behaved that way towards Suzy too and had no reason to be shy of her. She exhibited what I identified as an "aloof" personality, a concept from psychology which is widely recognised, although there were various differences in terminology between sources. Essentially, she made people have to exert an effort to engage with her. The concept was that an energy existed between any two people who were conversing, and that each person adopted a strategy to win the energy tug of war between them, and thus gain from the encounter. The concept identified four personality types, which were Intimidator, Inquisitor, Aloof and Poor Me, and psychologists identified that in any interaction, people tended to adopt one of these, and the other person adopted the opposite persona. People could change from one stance to another, depending upon who they were interacting with, but usually each individual had one predominant persona. In the case of Aloof, they required the other person to invest energy in making headway with a conversation by being monosyllabic, or reticent, and thus the other person felt drained by the encounter. Following the theory, this other person was likely to adopt the Inquisitor role, and question activities, motives etc. and Suzy often seemed to end up doing this but then became exhausted by the effort of trying to get Mary to engage in a conversation that she did not want to have. Eventually she would just give up trying, which was just what Mary wanted.

I knew the principles of these interpersonal dynamics from managing consultations with a variety of different patients and was aware that the only way to "win" in these situations, was not to play the game and to disengage, pointing out what the other person was doing and asking why they were being like that or returning to the subject when the other person approached because they then wanted something. That could then become the basis for negotiation.

The second thing was her habit of failing to tell the truth, either by omission or outright lying. To me this was easily spotted as there were always inconsistencies in her story and timeline of events, or material evidence. Examples of the latter included dust present on supposedly dusted surfaces, and bags of empty bottles in the recycling or in her car when she was adamant that she had not had people over to the house in our absence. However, the pattern was clear, and Mary would stick resolutely to her story in the sure and certain knowledge that Suzy would eventually accept it as the truth, simply because she did not want to believe that her daughter would lie to her or did not have the energy to pursue the conversation against the stonewall tactics Mary deployed. She would then defend that position against me.

Mary had lost her own father some 11 years earlier and so she and Suzy had, of necessity, managed as a team ever since. The idea that one half of the team would be less than honest to the other was simply not to be countenanced by Suzy, although Mary seemed to have no problem with it, mostly because it got her what she wanted without consequences. I would point out the inconsistencies, show Suzy the detail, but she would simply refuse to believe it and turn her wrath upon me instead for daring to suggest it. I learned just to keep quiet and do what I could to ameliorate the damage and highlight the worst of things. Mary's tendency to help herself to whatever she wanted of other people's things was similarly ignored by Suzy at first, but it became impossible for her to continue to do that. The level of Suzy's expensive perfume would drop, and there would be a waft of it lingering after Mary had left the house. She was not sparing with it either, appearing to spray a dense cloud of it which she would then walk through, rather than carefully apply it to strategic areas. There was also some obvious soiling and damage to some of Suzy's clothes which became noticeable, as Mary's clumsiness was notorious and, despite promises to be careful, red wine and food stains appeared on delicate silk garments, some of which had been borrowed with Suzy's knowledge, some of them without. Eventually Suzy asked me to put a lock on her built-in wardrobe, which I did. However, this was only ever used when we were staying away from the house, and Mary clearly continued to peruse Suzy's wardrobe at her leisure and would then sidle up to her mother before a social engagement to ask about an outfit to wear by saying "do you have anything like…" and then accurately describe an exact item in Suzy's wardrobe that she had identified on an earlier reconnaissance as the one she wanted to wear. Again, the subterfuge was clearly apparent to me, but Suzy either never tumbled it or was prepared to indulge her daughter.

The other thing that gained a lock was the drinks cabinet. I had felt that levels of spirits and sherry were unaccountably dropping for some time, but there was one evening when Suzy and I went out for a meal and Mary had a girlfriend over. They were to share a bottle of prosecco which they had purchased, and when we returned, they saluted our return by raising their glasses, showing the contents to be the brownest prosecco I had ever seen. Fearing the worst, I checked the cabinet, only to find half of my cognac gone, no doubt used as a mixer to make the prosecco a little more interesting. When questioned about this raiding of my brandy to liven up their fizz though, the girls naturally denied it and drained their glasses to remove any evidence. I fitted the lock the next day.

Mary was a great one too for finishing things up, or rather, not quite. She clearly never wanted to be accused of doing this, so she would eat whatever it was down to the last teaspoonful and then leave this in the container, be it ice cream, chocolate spread, anything. Left-over pie would have the filling excavated away leaving a large overhang of pastry, whilst chocolate cake would lose icing from the top, and the filling between the sponge layers would develop a concave surface, like pointing between courses of brickwork, where Mary would have run her finger along to scoop some out to transfer to her mouth and remove by sucking. I did not like to think about how many times that sucked finger had been reapplied to the filling for subsequent loads. The only exception to this rule of not quite finishing stuff was soft drinks of which she would drink the house dry without telling anybody so that there were none available if we went to offer one to a guest.

Almost entirely due to the efforts of Mary, we did not own a whole set of drinking glasses at all. This was usually due to clumsiness augmented by her infuriating habit of insisting on marking her time at home by the carrying of a recently filled hot water bottle under one arm at all times. I never really identified where this habit had come from, or why Mary failed to just put on warmer clothing, but it was a habit that seemed oblivious of ambient or external temperature, current clothing, or time of year. It had to be admitted that Suzy herself had something of a hot water bottle habit, but Mary took it to a whole new level. The central heating might be set high enough to grow exotic flora within the lounge, but Mary would refill her bottle at least hourly, at considerable wastage of water and electricity, to my mind.

The latest glass to bite the dust was one of our best Villeroy and Boch set, which Mary had decided was the only thing suitable from which she could quaff the contents of her 2.5 litre box of supermarket dry white, despite there being many alternatives available, including some waifs and strays from previous sets whose numbers had been similarly depleted. The glass in question was on its third refill when it succumbed to the combination of poor dexterity, caused by the clasping of the hot water bottle, and the sleeve of a dressing gown that was both capacious and inadequately supervised. The usual sullen response of absence of personal blame and insincere promises of replacement followed, the latter being a strategy that was adopted when guilt was so obvious that even Mary felt she could not deny it. At least, that was the last breakage that I was certain of. Recently I had begun to suspect another casualty was my favourite pint glass that Mary had used every night for her nocturnal water supply for several years. I had brought it back from the West Country with me some ten years previously, and it sported an illustration on the front of a surfboard being held upright by a fellow wearing the unlikely combination of a monk's habit and wayfarer sunglasses. His feet were encased in sandals which, I had to concede, could have gone with either of the other two items mentioned, though possibly not both. Certainly, the glass' absence had gone unremarked upon by its usual user, who had taken to purloining her mother's favourite such glass instead.

Mary was a "boomerang child", to use the current parlance for those who had flown the nest only to return. In fact, this was currently her third return, so she was less like a boomerang and more like a yo-yo. She had initially gone to university, though had spent more and more time back at home during the second year, and hardly seemed to be going there at all in her third whilst writing her dissertation. She then returned home whilst starting work as a teaching assistant in an infant's school, which she was clearly very good at and had a natural aptitude for, but which offered no career path or chance of promotion. She moved out into a flat with a friend but came back after only six months. She then had a serious relationship with a boy she had met when they were both training to be Police Special Constables, and they got as far as buying a house together, but that relationship had unfortunately fallen apart, and she was now back home again. Despite having apparently run a home herself, and gained some insight into the difficulties of living with someone who had many of the same character traits as herself, she seemed to bring none of this to bear upon her return to the family home, and instead she lapsed into the previous habit of waiting for meals to be provided, laundry to be done, and texting her mother downstairs to request that Suzy relinquish the comforts of the lounge in order to bring a hot chocolate up to her bedroom, a request which Suzy invariably complied with to my horror. I found it ironic that Mary found the character of Stacey so annoying in the BBC programme "Gavin and Stacey" because Stacey was so self-centred and needy, but she apparently had no insight into the fact that her own character was not too dissimilar. Whilst Mary found it hard to say no to others who asked things of her, she found it all too easy to say this to her mother and did not put herself forward to offer anything at home unasked. In the whole year that she lived in her own house, we were only asked over once for a meal, but there were several requests for us to visit for more practical input requiring cleaning skills or a toolkit, or for me to level the small back garden and seed it with grass for a lawn.

It was much the same pattern on her return to the family home. Regardless of how late Suzy and I worked, or how busy we were, although Mary finished work at four o'clock in the afternoon we never returned to the sounds and smells of a meal underway, but, instead, the inevitable enquiry from Mary as to what we would be cooking that evening that she might share. She had also retained the habit of going out to nightclubs which meant that Suzy and I were woken at three or four o'clock in the morning by noise, light, and general chaos as an inebriated Mary got herself ready for bed, absolutely certain in herself that she was making no more noise than a mouse in carpet slippers. But woe betide Suzy, or I, if we made any noise getting up and ready for work just an hour or so later.

She did, however, have many laudable traits too. She always won praise at work for her dedication and industry and was popular wherever she went, making friends and forming close bonds with colleagues. When she worked in the Pre-Primary School as a teaching assistant, the pupils and staff alike were devastated when she left. The same occurred in her next role at the local university where she effortlessly seemed to span the gulf between the students and the faculty staff as she was so much closer in age to the former and understood their issues so well but was part of the latter team. From there she joined the police and won plaudits for her attention to detail in the safeguarding cases that she worked on. Whenever her behaviour was highlighted against her work ethic, she would say that she did not see the need to bother because this was her home where she should be able to relax. We would point out that it was our home too, but we were busy keeping it going and could not afford to sit in front of the television all day wearing a onesie, cuddling a hot water bottle, and drinking vats of over-sweetened tea, but Mary merely shrugged this off. She clearly felt that it was our job to make her life as easy as possible.

Part of the difficulty that I felt was that I never really knew what my role was in her life. As she had been without her father for so many years, there was no clash and I found myself in the father role within the household, but I never really felt that this was how Mary viewed me and she certainly did not afford me the respect that a father might feel was his due. She did not seem to feel that I had any authority over her and so, with Suzy being at best ambivalent over authority herself, tending to back down when push came to shove, and not giving me any support against Mary, I felt as if I was little more than a spectator in my own home. As the years passed, she formed another relationship and moved away to Essex to set up home with that new partner. They came back fairly regularly, and I noticed that she started to fall less readily into the old patterns of behaviour whenever she came home to stay, but I always wished that she had applied the same level of dedication to the issues we had at home as she had done with her work. That whole situation went on much too long for my liking and I was relieved when Mary finally left. It was lovely to subsequently find, after a year or two of managing her own place, that we got on better when she visited thereafter.

CHAPTER 21

It is amazing just how quickly a relationship can change, and this one changed almost overnight, although we had rubbed along together, mostly under the same roof, for a dozen years or so. Sometimes things were smooth, at others a little more abrasive. She seemed to have accepted that I am a necessary part of her life, mostly because I have been married to her mother for nearly ten years now but has never seemed to find the right pigeonhole to put me into. I am useful to keep the fridge stocked and the house warm, but always seemed to serve no other purpose in her life except as an occasional taxi. She and her mother had formed a close-knit partnership in which Mary seemed to have the upper hand, having learned quite early on that being brattish and sulky generally seemed to get her what she wanted and kept her mother off her back. She also picked up on the fact that her mother would defend her against me, even if what I thought should happen was clearly what Suzy thought should happen. She just would never side with me against her daughter. And so, the animosity ebbed and flowed over the years, slowly seeming to improve with the passing of years and her leaving home, but never really feeling comfortable. And then came that Christmas.

I did not routinely communicate directly with Mary unless it was face-to-face and so I picked up the details from my discussions with Suzy. She related that Mary was fed up down in Essex because her clothes were not fitting her and she did not seem to be able to shift this bit of weight that she had put on, despite dieting and exercising vigorously. Suzy asked if I could just check things over when Mary came to stay for Christmas from Essex with her partner, James, and I agreed to do that. They arrived on Christmas Eve and so I was pressed into service quite quickly, and the first thing I noticed was that Mary had a bit of a bulgy tummy whilst the rest of her still looked slim. The mantra in medical school, and ever since, was that all women of child-bearing age are pregnant until proven otherwise, but Mary was university educated and very sharp in most things, so I presumed that she had already considered and excluded that possibility. Examination of her tummy showed a distinct bulge arising from the pelvis, and my mind ran through the list of Fs that one is meant to consider in cases of abdominal distension – Fat, Fluid, Faeces, Flatus, Foetus. There it was again, and if I have learnt anything through a long career it is that one should never assume anything, and so I asked if there was any chance at all that she might be pregnant. Well, I got chapter and verse about how busy she and James were, never had any time for that sort of thing, how she had stopped her pill about a year ago as it made her feel crap, and she hadn't had a period in all that time, and as for sex! Haley's comet appeared more frequently! Well, there had possibly been three occasions in that whole year. I pointed out that once would have been enough and that, whilst post-pill amennorhoea is a common phenomenon, it would have masked whether or not she was actually ovulating so it was still possible and perhaps a pregnancy test would be a good idea. Clearly the shops were not open again until Boxing Day, but she was straight round there for one once they were. If the test strip had an area saying, "Oh My God, you are *so* pregnant", then this is the one that would have been highlighted. As it was it practically shouted the result PREGNANT, at which point Mary's jaw hit the floor. This was definitely not on her "things to do" list, despite her being nearly thirty. There was plenty of time for kids later, she said, and yet it seemed that fate had dealt her a joker in the pack. And she was quite well gone too. The size of her uterine swelling suggested that she was into her fifth month, so things needed to be arranged fast. She was the envy of some of her friends who had experienced torrid pregnancies and wondered how she could not have known, let alone what her secret was to avoid even a shred of morning sickness. Prosecco was suggested as the reason by Mary but was unlikely to be taken seriously. Needless to say, that ruined her festivities as she immediately transferred to sparkling water with elderflower cordial and started researching what she needed to do once back at Essex. What she discovered was that her local hospital had a CQC rating and patient experience feedback that would have been depressing for a war zone, and so it was decided that she would relocate back to Norfolk and have the baby there, going back to Essex once baby was three or four weeks old. And so, this is what she did, making endless arrangements, continuing to work remotely as she had done throughout the covid-19 pandemic, and having all of her antenatal care locally, whilst we rearranged her room to allow it to accommodate the baby, with changing station, cot, pram, and the many other accoutrements that new mum's simply must have. Once she had got over the surprise and adjusted to her new reality, she was like a changed person. Focused and determined, keeping everything together, researching endlessly, checking out social media sites, and developing into a blooming expectant mum. Throughout this time, her attitude towards me thawed immensely and we got on so much better. I did not think I had really done anything amazing to bring this about. If anything, I had been the harbinger of news that was apparently unwanted at the time, but our whole relationship changed for the better.

Because she had presented late, well past the usual time for a dating scan, the scanners could not be sure of her due date because the algorithms for size and gestation were less accurate at that stage of pregnancy. Mary could though, as there was only one possible assignation with James that could have caused this end result in the time frame, but the hospital team planned to take Mary in on her due date to induce delivery as they could not be sure that she would not be post-term and thus risk placental function declining to the baby's detriment. Therefore, on the appointed day she awaited the summons, only to be told late in the day that there were no beds available, and she would have to wait. Fortunately, the decks were sufficiently cleared for her to attend the following evening and a pessary was administered to get things going. Nothing much happened that first night, but she was kept awake by a lady in the next bed who was obviously in considerable discomfort but having to cope with it alone, partners not being allowed on the ward except during visiting hours, which were long since over. This lady had progressed and moved to the delivery floor by the next day, at which point she could be accompanied, and Mary was pleased with the relief from that noise, but the daily hustle and bustle of the ward prevented her from getting any sleep that day. The pessary began to have its effect and was topped up by a second dose that evening, by which time Mary realized that she had now become the noisy woman in pain in the next bed.

The call came at three in the morning that Mary was being moved to the delivery floor and so James could come up to join her. Not being a driver himself, that involved one of us taking him and so Suzy kindly volunteered as I was at work the next day. Dispatches on progress were sent throughout the day, culminating in the safe delivery of a baby boy late in the evening. Although things had progressed nicely at first, the baby had decided to roll onto his back on the way down, causing a mismatch between his head dimensions and the birth canal, such that he had to be helped out into the world by a suction machine that attached to the scalp and sucked in a mushroom-shaped bulge of it to allow traction without compression. His head looked a bit odd for a couple of days afterwards, and Mary needed a cut to ease the egress of boy and machine part, but otherwise all was well.

James was in awe of how Mary had coped with it all, and Mary just seemed to ooze competent motherhood from every pore. She took everything in her stride, clearly applied her learning to events that unfolded for both her and her newborn son, and never seemed flustered. Once home, feeding and other routines developed quickly and she just seemed like somebody who had been waiting for this thing to happen in her life, without ever knowing it. Again, her relationship with me just seemed to find another gear. It might have helped that she had the confidence of doctor on call at any hour of the day or night, and it probably helped that she had the opportunity to bond with her baby without having to attend to running a house, cooking, cleaning, shopping or any of the other many duties that face most new mothers on their return home, but whatever it was, we just got on. It was simple, it was natural, we dealt with each other differently, and it reminded me of how things had been with my own daughters back in the day, before everything turned shitty, and it has continued in this vein ever since. She even bought us a lovely set of glasses for our anniversary. Clearly, the "hang in there and wait for a change in the weather" approach worked, but it was a long time coming.

CHAPTER 22

So back to practice, and the bastard who had denied me my final hours with my father eventually decided it was time to retire. I was pleased to see him gone but that did leave me to manage the practice alone whilst seeking a replacement. Unfortunately, the tide had turned on General Practice and it was far from the appealing and over-subscribed profession that it had been when I started out. There were several elements to this, but I had witnessed the trend throughout my career. The main problem was that Primary Care had become the dumping ground for everything that the hospital departments no longer wanted to do, and much of this was down to an ever-increasing workload on them without the resources to manage it. When I was young, our GP was a single-handed guy who worked out of two rooms in his own house with his wife acting as receptionist. Patients simply turned up and sat and waited until they were seen, and the doctor did everything, from dressings and injections to diagnosis and syringing out ears. In order to make some extra money this GP also acted as police surgeon and so was regularly called away from surgery at which point his wife would say that he was likely to be out for some time and would we mind coming back tomorrow. Actually, we mostly would mind but had little choice. If any blood tests were needed, and these were rare, we were given a form to take to the local hospital where the blood would be taken. When I sat in on outpatient clinics as a student it was common to find patients being referred with a letter that said something like "I believe this patient may have asthma/ high blood pressure / insert other simply managed condition here, and I would be grateful if you would kindly see them and treat accordingly." Therefore, clinics had a lot of this type of work to do and then went on seeing patients regularly for months or years afterwards. Two main things that happened is that more patients started getting long term conditions, and fewer people died of them. There may have been an increase in life expectancy over the years, but the time gained is often not spent in good health. The outpatient workload became too much and so it was dumped onto the GP service to do instead, without any consideration on how this would be managed or any transfer of funding with which to do it. The best analogy that I can think of is a juggler. You may watch him balancing on a unicycle and juggling three rings and think that this was pretty difficult, and had taken time and practice to achieve, and be impressed to start with. This could well be the GP at the start. Imagine then that the hospital acts like the juggler's assistant and starts throwing him extra rings which he has to incorporate into what he is doing, until at last he is balancing on the unicycle and juggling nine rings. An impressive feat, but not one that he can do for long, and he is glad when the warm and appreciative applause of the audience gives him his cue to hand back the rings and dismount. Unfortunately, the GP does not have that option. Firstly, there is no warm and appreciative applause for managing the feat of more and more work on the same resources, just the sound of somebody hunting around for more rings to throw in his direction. Secondly, there is no dismount option. The only way to manage the workload is to delegate, hence the introduction of nurses who have special training to allow them to follow protocols to manage long term conditions, with the GP retaining overall responsibility. The GP must employ these nurses at his own expense in order to do the work that he did not ask for and was not paid for. Increasing workload has meant an expansion of ancillary clinical staff so that many practices now number amongst their staff roles such as phlebotomist, health care assistant, nurse, specialist nurse, advanced nurse practitioner, paramedic, physiotherapist and counsellor. To back up all of these there are expanded reception, secretarial and data input staff. From the GP staff of one that I saw in my youth, the average GP will now have six or more whole time equivalent staff to help him manage the practice workload. But despite all of these extra staff, we are still left on the unicycle and with more hoops than we had at the outset. And this is just the clinical workload. Practices are essentially small businesses and so there are the added burdens of dealing with staff, accounts, cashflow, premises, and dispensing if the practice can dispense medications to its own patients. All of this has to be dealt with as well and demands all sorts of meetings as well as time for patient contact. Increasingly this is seen as too much to manage, especially as the financial rewards have been dropping for more than a decade and the financial commitment to being a partner have become significant.

Over two years I had two prospective partners start but fail to complete their probation periods for one reason or another. They would have been OK as salaried doctors or under somebody else's supervision but not as stand-alone practitioners. At last, I did find a new partner, who was fine through his probation, but before the ink was dry on the partnership agreement, he showed that he had a completely new agenda regarding ways of the practice making money, some of which were barely legal. I found I did not have the stomach for the fight and left. It may well have been that I was just not temperamentally suited to partnership as I had not had a happy time at all.

I now work as a salaried doctor, just concentrating on the clinical aspects of work and being an employee so I have none of the other issues to deal with, and I much prefer it. I wish that I had discovered that earlier in my career as I might have been more content, but it was not such an easy option back then. Now practices are crying out for salaried doctors as they cannot attract partners, so it seems that I am not alone. Who knows what the future holds in that direction, and what will happen if nobody wants to be a partner any longer?

But work is still busy enough on its own. The number of complicated patients with multiple morbidities has increased dramatically, as have their potential treatments. These will not be every patient, but they take up a lot of our time. The average GP has a list size of 1800 patients, and a good few hundred of these will be complex to deal with. We are given appointments that are ten minute long, but it can take almost that length of time to read through the records to remind ourselves of a patient's past and recent medical history and their medications, read relevant recent hospital letters and test results, and feel comfortable with the current context of this consultation, even before the consultation starts. And there might be forty or so of these in a day as well as all of the administration that goes with it, such as documenting the consultation, arranging tests and investigations, dictating letters etc., as well as all the incoming results and clinic letters. At the end of a ten-hour day, I am done, and I drag what is left of me back to my home and family. I work alternate days and the only way I can get through a day sometimes is the knowledge that I am not working on the following day. If I did not have that reassuring break, then at the end of Monday night I would consider it an impossibly high mountain to climb to get to the end of the week. Perhaps when I was younger, I may have managed better, but as I am now in my sixties the fact that I am working at all means that if I were an animal I would be considered as "critically endangered" as so few GPs of my age are still in that position. In not many years' time that designation will change to "at risk of extinction". General Practice seems to be a young person's game now just to manage the workload, but this comes at the risk of losing a wealth of experience and knowledge. The profession is already finding it hard to attract new GPs and retain those that it has. I can see no strategy in place to change this situation, but I hope that it does not get to the point where there is just a stampede for the door.

CHAPTER 23

It was not just Mary who had produced offspring that I became involved with. After much sleep lost to turmoil and fruitless reflection, I had resigned myself several years previously to the fact that I was unlikely to be a part of the lives of any of my children, or of any grandchildren that may come along in due course. Like my other two children, my eldest daughter, Rose, had absented herself from my life for some nine years following my divorce from their mother and I had seen no indication that anything would change about that. However, a text message from Rose had come to me unexpectedly one February, with an antenatal ultrasound image attached and it contained the message that she hoped that I would be involved with my first grandchild as I "had already missed so much." Is not that the truth, I thought, though it had not been my own choice. I thought through a silent rollcall of missed significant life events, including the marriage of Rose and her husband, Jackson barely eighteen months before. I had been aware of it, of course, having managed to find some on-line existence of each of my children and glean snippets of their lives from that, lives whose content and development had been lost to me for so long. I had identified the date and time of the ceremony, and had a good punt at the likely venue, which turned out to have been accurate, but I would never have considered turning up un-invited. It was their big day after all, and it was not for me to attempt to enforce a reconciliation that was highly likely to have remained unwanted after so many years. However, I did rue missing out on the period of happy anticipation before the event, being able to give her away in the ceremony, the loss of the father-daughter dance, and the father of the bride speech which is really just a chance for the father to repay with embarrassment all the occasions that his daughter has embarrassed or inconvenienced him until that point in their lives. I regretted the apparent waste of all those childhood events that I had secreted away in my memory as the years passed, thinking that they would make ideal content for the speech that I had one day hoped to make.

For instance, there was the occasion when I had taken her swimming when she can have been no more than four or five years old. Due to her lack of independence at that age I had, of necessity, to share a changing cubicle with her. After getting her dry, talcum powdered, and dressed, I had to attempt to get myself dried and dressed in a suitably discrete fashion by keeping myself covered with the towel as much as possible and donning underwear whilst that article was still draped around me. I had thought that I was doing a reasonable job of this, an illusion that was duly shattered when I heard her pipe up, with devastating clarity that the rest of the changing room surely must have heard

"I haven't got one of those, have I Daddy?"

From previous experience, I knew that any attempts at hushing up the subject never worked and only led to further questioning. I was therefore forced to try to hurry through the rest of my changing just get out of there, struggling to pull my clothing on over damp skin to which it clung and rolled up, hampering the task and my attempts to do it quickly. Swimming with Rose was a regular event as her mother, my first wife, Rebekah, did not "do" swimming. This aversion was for no apparent or explained reason, like so much else that she chose to absent herself from, but she had been clear about the aspiration that she wanted Rose to learn how to swim, as did I. I had not learned to swim until I was into my teens and knew the many missed opportunities with friends and family that this had led to, and I did not want Rose to similarly miss out.

There was also the episode when Rose was a year or two older and was going through a typical childhood fascination with the abundance of insect life to be found in our garden in the Norfolk countryside. Having found several different examples one sunny summer afternoon, she decided she would like to study bugs when she was older, in much the same way that I remembered that I had espoused the idea of becoming a bus conductor after my first trip on a red double-decker as a child during which I was fascinated by the machine that dispensed the tickets. In those days, the machine had been slung around the neck of the conductor against a short leather apron, rather than perched on the edge of a counter next to the driver. The conductor had even given me the end of the ticket roll to keep at the end of the trip. When I asked Rose what this study of bugs might be called, she gave it careful thought for a moment and declared it to be "Buggery!" in the same clear and authoritative tone I remembered from the swimming pool incident. And there were so many more, now all just wasted material, though fond memories none the less.

Perhaps the worst part of this whole situation for me was that I could not help feeling just a bit relieved, and I still feel incredibly guilty about that. I am fairly sure that the duties of hosting a wedding would tax my social abilities up to, if not beyond, their limit. This would have been made worse by having no idea what any of the company present thought of or expected from me because Rose's mother would have got her oar in first. Part of her control was always propaganda, making sure she got her version of events in first, so anybody else had to contradict that and convince the listener of this new version over the one that they had already heard. And you can be sure that everybody present would have been given her story and had it repeated several times. When I eventually got to meet Jackson's family, it was clear from their response that I was nothing like the person they expected me to be.

I could probably have managed the wedding speech by treating it as a lecture, playing a role if you will. But I have seen friends manage their own daughters' weddings, being effortlessly charming with the friends of the bride, one of the lads with the groom's entourage, discussing cricket and football knowledgeably, perhaps breaking the ice before the big day with a round of golf, and just breezing through the day full of *bon homie* and good red wine. None of that is within my capabilities.

I would attempt to get through it, of course, but it is likely that the two most common comments during the day would be "Doesn't the bride look lovely" and "Has anybody seen John?" Now I hear that my other daughter is soon to be married, without me again, and I have that same feeling of sorrow and relief in equal measure, with a giant side order of guilt for thinking that way.

The missed wedding was just the latest of several missed events. When Rose went to university I had been excluded and had subsequently missed settling her in, hearing about her university life, sports clubs, nights out, teaching placements etc. and had missed watching her mature and grow in self-confidence. Instead, I had to console myself with the crumbs I managed to glean from social media and other sources. Of course, I was not invited to the graduation ceremony after she had passed with a 2:1 degree, and neither was I involved in her finding gainful employment in her chosen profession, or consoling her as real life and its multitude of unexpected responsibilities set in. Once the date of the wedding had passed without any contact from her, I just believed that the obvious time for her to have reached out to me had gone, and I was therefore unlikely to be allowed into her life again. There had been a tentative exchange of texts the previous year before the engagement had been announced, but it was apparent that there was still uncertainty on both sides, and the attempt had foundered. However, I remained as much in the dark as ever about exactly what I had supposed to have done to deliver such behaviour upon myself.

When the breakthrough in communications came, there had been a tacit agreement that neither party would "go there" as far as the past went, and so the reasons for the long estrangement remained the elephant in the room each time we met, albeit an elephant that did seem to diminish in size and importance with each occasion. But I had decided that if that was the price that I had to pay for having a relationship with my daughter and grandson, then so be it. Having attained my late fifties, pragmatism had become my byword and I no longer harboured expectations. Perhaps I should have done, and pursued them more vigorously, but I also believed that sometimes you just need to settle for what you have and be grateful for it. When Mary gave birth, Rose had already produced two boys, Augustus and Luke, and we had seen them several times, and I was receiving almost daily updates and photos from her. However, things have never got back to the point that they were previously at. Part of the reason for that is me keeping Rose at arm's length as that elephant remains in the room, however small. Her mother had cheated on me, lied about that and other things consistently, and tried to imply that I had a chance of reconciliation in order to manipulate the separation and get more concessions and money from me. I had never asked the children to choose between, us, but they did, probably at their mother's insistence. And they chose her, the liar, the cheat, the manipulator. If that was their choice, then what must they have thought of me? This is another issue that remains unresolved. That, and the absence of apology or explanation for the separation. It really doesn't feel like it should, but I am determined to maintain a relationship with my grandsons. I remember the first Christmas after Augustus had been born in the Summer. I sat at my ease with my grandson on my knee and I felt something akin to contentment. As recently as a year previously I could not have considered that eventuality to be possible , and yet, there I was, with him seated happily on my lap. The young lad was enchanted by the twinkling Christmas tree lights and was dressed in pyjamas with a bright holly motif but remained happily ignorant of the mounting excitement of everyone else around him as his First Christmas rapidly approached. I had enquired as to what would be a suitable and welcome gift for my grandson and had been informed by Rose about the desired combination of seat and activity table that she and her husband had in mind for him. This had been duly purchased and sat, carefully wrapped but bulky and obvious in its box, beneath the be-decked Christmas tree in my daughter's sitting room. A token gift was also there for my daughter and son-in-law. An olive branch had been offered and I had grasped it gratefully and did not wish to seem churlish or petty.

Suzy and I, Suzy having been my wife of six years by then, had been over to my daughter and son-in-law's home in the preceding months, both throughout the pregnancy and since the birth, and we had been invited to come earlier that day to enjoy cuddles and games with the young lad, who had then observed us all enjoying our evening meal from the vantage point of his highchair. Following the meal, we had been involved with his nightly bath time routine. He had lain there, chubbily splashing the water with his thrashing legs, and laughing up at us with his infectious giggle. I was now engaged in the final cuddle which preceded the bed-time bottle and subsequent putting to bed, and Augustus exuded the faint scent of lavender from the "bed-time" talc that had been applied after drying with a towel that had been warmed on the radiator. He sat there happily enough, occasionally rubbing a tired eye with the back of a chubby hand. He is now four and has been joined by his younger brother, Luke, now two years old.

I had tested the water with my own mother since being back in touch with Rose, but it was clear that she had no interest in Rose or her latest great-grandchildren after the way that myself and both she and my father had been treated, so I was not going to push that at all. I could see how much my mother had been hurt by the omission and that she felt the same for Dad who had not had the chance of a reconciliation himself before he had been taken. I could not use their experiences as a yardstick for what it was like to be a grandfather and so I looked back at memories of my own grandparents.

I only remembered those on my maternal side. Dad's father had died before Steve and I were born, and his mother died before we were two years old. She had apparently seen us once as babies, but that was it, and I obviously have no recollection of that meeting. So, I only really remember my mother's parents, known to us as Nana and Grandpa.

My first memories of them are at the guest house that they ran on the south coast. Grandpa had been a career soldier in the Royal Artillery and had been involved in organising air defences along the south coast in the second world war, and at the time of my first memories he was then still working in defence at the south coast docks near to where they lived. They had bought two adjacent properties and made alterations so that together they formed the guest house, but I realise now that I had not really understood everything about that arrangement at the time. I remember that my bedroom door had a number on it every time that we stayed with them, and that this seemed somewhat at odds with my usual experience of bedroom doors in other people's houses. Also, I remember that each morning we had to go through a room full of people sitting at small tables and eating when we went down for breakfast as a family, with us sitting with Nana and Grandpa at a separate table beyond a curtain. Also, all the cereals were in large plastic containers with pop-up flaps in the lid, rather than the scrunched down packets inside boxes that I was used to at home. The reasons for this only became clear later.

They also had a dog, of whom I was a little afraid, even though he was only a small poodle. In fact, considering how much dogs became an integral part of my adult life, it seems strange that I was so afraid of them as a child. This dog was so full of joy and play that he was named "Gayboy", a name that raised no eyebrows in those days, but which would probably do so nowadays. Certainly not the sort of thing that could easily be called across a playing field without some puzzled stares or somebody taking offence. The poodle seemed to spend his nights in the summerhouse in the back garden and then be let out to play each morning, with daily walks at some point.

I remember walks around the boating lake in the nearby park, and that us two boys had a model sailing boat that we could float across the water, although it had no motor so the prevailing wind, or lack of it, did much to control whether the boat ended up at the opposite bank or stranded in the middle, and the boat unfortunately did not last too long. There was certainly no chance of a radio-controlled version. I also remember being bitten on the thumb by a swan when I was too slow to dole out the stale bread that we habitually took with us to the park for feeding purposes. Down the road, some ten minutes' walk away, was the shingle beach leading to the pier over on the right, which supported some fairground rides and a small rollercoaster and from the base of which small hovercraft would set off across the Solent, heading for the Isle of Wight, or "Widgit" as my father would always pronounce it. That was just one of his phrases, like "I have had enough sufficientness," and "some say Good Old John, others tell the truth!" I was terrified of the hovercraft because I could not tolerate the enormous amount of noise they generated, and so I covered my ears and hid behind the pier buildings whenever one started up the engine, whose note rose in pitch and volume until it was practically screaming, at which point it rose up on its skirt before sliding effortlessly sideways into the water, scattering shingle from the beach as it went. From the beach one could also see the strangely sinister brick-built forts, dating from the Napoleonic wars, in the water beyond. These always looked slightly frightening, which was not at all helped when they acted as the setting for an episode of Dr Who involving sea monsters.

The beach did reluctantly yield some sand as the tide receded and this proved much more fun for Steve and me with buckets and spades at the ready. I can remember a time when we thought we had uncovered a treasure hoard, for wherever we dug on that morning, we found the odd three-penny or sixpence piece, this being well before decimalisation of the currency. We dug for ages, uncovering several shillings worth of small change, and never noticed that Nana and Grandpa, seated nearby in their folding picnic chairs, and encouraging us in our efforts, were surreptitiously tossing the coins in at odd moments for us to find as if newly uncovered.

Then suddenly the guest house was no more, and my grandparents had moved into a modern bungalow along the coast, and it is this house and my grandparents' time within it that I remember the most. I later found that the move was enforced because Grandpa had emphysema, for both he and Nana were long-term smokers, and his health had deteriorated so that they could no longer manage the guest house. I do remember Grandpa not moving around so much and frequently coughing and spitting into tissues which accumulated at his chairside, but these were swiftly moved away from us children once noticed, and their significance was lost on the us at the time.

The bungalow had a stone frontage and large sweeping wrap-around front garden with low retainer wall, as it was situated on the corner of two roads. My memories of this house are of venetian blinds at every window, internal doors that locked, with the door to the lounge and kitchen being mostly glass, and a small sunroom behind the garage, with shelves of plants along the glass wall to the right, and a red and white striped fly screen at the sliding door. This door led out to the back yard which contained a shed-cum-summerhouse that had that wonderful smell of warm cedar wood and contained the deckchairs and windbreaks that were a vital part of any trip to the British seaside. There were also bowls of mints around the lounge, and we would attempt to sneak these from time to time although this was not encouraged. There seemed to me at that age, a strange association between being older and having a fondness for peppermints that I could never quite fathom, and I have not yet succumbed to that affliction. On the walls of the hall of the bungalow, and in a couple of cabinets nearby, were exotica from foreign travels, such as beaten metalwork, a curved dagger in a sheath, and various bowls and ornaments. There was also an exotic-looking shallow bowl that contained a cactus plant growing in a special compost that crunched when it was pressed and, no doubt, gave the sharp drainage that the plant required. The cactus was spiny, and Steve and I would carefully see if we could insert a small finger between the spines to touch the firm fleshy stem without getting impaled, with one eye on the other twin to ensure no sudden jog of the elbow at an inopportune moment.

The kitchen was relatively small, much smaller than that of the guest house, yet had a huge fridge with a lockable door and thick sides. Opposite this was the biggest gas cooker I had ever seen, with several rings and a warming plate as well as several doors at the front. On the wall over the sink was a plastic canister holding loose tea, with a button on the front that one pushed to dispense a spoonful of tea into a warmed teapot when a brew was required, with Nana insisting on one spoon for each person and one for the pot. On the worktop near the serving hatch through to the dining room, was a small coffee grinder with an open top for pouring in coffee beans, a handle on the side which was turned to grind the beans, and a pull-out drawer which would collect the ground coffee to be then tipped into the percolator. This would be transferred to sit silently on the sideboard in the dining room until it started to gloop and hiss to signify that coffee was now ready for the grown-ups.

The bungalow was not too far from the New Forest, whose tendrils crept well beyond its boundary so that there seemed to be mature trees everywhere around the estate where the bungalow was situated. Steve and I shared a twin room when we stayed at the bungalow, the two beds separated by the width of a bedside unit made of dark wood, containing an in-built clock with luminous hands and numbers. We spent many wet days on holiday there pretending to have wars by each hiding behind a bed, as if in a trench, and trying to hit the other with elastic bands fired across the no-man's-land in between, bobbing our heads up and down slightly to draw fire so that we could then straighten up ourselves and let loose with our own shot.

There was one regular aspect of staying there as a family which did not really become apparent to me until I was much older. Our parents were always early risers, and my father would like to take an early morning walk when in Dorset, whilst Mum stayed around in case she was needed to help, being very aware of how much intrusion we must have caused to her parents' usual routine. Steve and I usually accompanied Dad, and we would stop in at the Little Chef cafeteria situated in a small service station at a roundabout nearby, and we would have tea or orange juice and hot buttered toast. We considered this to be quite a treat. Mum would later say that this was a waste of money as we could have breakfast once we got back, and we usually did go on to have cereal or something extra, but Dad kept on doing it. I later realised that this must have been a special time for him, a time to have his sons to himself and be at his leisure for a short while. As I have mentioned earlier, he worked long hours and had a long commute at each end of the day involving at least two buses each way and he had little time off with few holidays. This was an opportunity to have quality time with his sons, and if such time was to be spent on a stroll in the morning sunshine and with hot buttered toast, then so be it. We seemed to talk about everything under the sun, and he would point things out as we walked and ask us about them or tell us things about those objects. He would also whistle or sing snatches of music hall songs, talk a little about his own childhood, tell awful jokes, and just seem relaxed. This was one time when we were not afraid to say or do the wrong thing, for he seemed to have all the time in the world for us, and it was our special thing to do. I just wish he could have been more like that for more of the time. Some children would crave excitement, rides on the pier, ice creams and candy floss, and we might ask for those too, but when I think back on it that time with our father on those summer morning strolls was special.

Although I can remember certain things about Grandpa from when I was very young, such as his trilby hat with a band around it, and him wearing cardigans, pastel-coloured socks, and brown Hush Puppy shoes, I did not notice anything much else at that age. However, as mentioned, he was ill with emphysema and heart failure, and so he was never robust. Although his lack of wind meant that he could not walk far or play ball games, he still liked to be involved with us children and he entertained Steve and I in several ways. There were magic tricks which he performed with the phrase "Gully, gully, gully, one two three!" instead of abracadabra, or anything similar, with a few small props from some ancient magic set. He made things seemingly disappear and reappear convincingly. There were also the unsuitable stories that he told, and which dated from his time in the Army. These were usually told at mealtimes and included subjects such as the various grisly findings left behind by the enemy as his unit advanced through the desert. These were received with horrified fascination by Steve and I, and loud "tutting" sounds from Mum and Nana who felt they were wholly unsuitable at any time, let alone when everyone was eating. He also showed us memorabilia from his army days, such as his regimental cap, and photos, and his regimental sword. Grandpa had also served in India and developed a particular liking for two things at meal-times – the first was mango chutney, a previously unheard-of luxury that we soon found equally enchanting, and easily recognised by the tall square jar with a green label and gold lettering. The other was a side relish, that seemed to be made of sliced and peeled cucumber with thinly sliced onion in a vinaigrette. There was always a small dish of this at Grandpa's elbow for every meal except breakfast and it was made clear that the Steve and I were not allowed to touch it.

Another realisation that came much later in life was how pleased Grandpa was with Steve and me. He and Nana had had three daughters of their own, and they had given them six granddaughters between them before we came along. He certainly seemed to relish having some boys in his life.

When Grandpa had been well enough to visit our family home, I remember that Nana had always done the driving, and that their departures were always accompanied by Grandpa waving a yellow duster vigorously from the passenger window, the duster primarily being there to wipe condensation from the inner surface of the windscreen. Grandpa died whilst on a trip to some relatives in the Northeast of England when I was only eleven, but these were the memories that stayed with me. In due course, I came into possession of Grandpa's sword. Not sharp, of course, but it was basket-hilted with a handle made of fine wire around a leather grip, and it was sheathed in a leather scabbard which bore a shiny patina from being handled. Time had left its tarnish on the blade so that some of the inscription there could not be read, and I always vowed to have it restored properly, but somehow, I have never got around to it, though the sword is up in the wardrobe even now.

Nana was a much stronger memory, mostly because she outlived Grandpa by some decades. She was a forthright and determined lady, who had learned to drive by first driving lorries during the Second World War and drove ever-after as if she was still surrounded by a surfeit of sturdy metal bodywork. She was not apparently incommoded by any potential difficulty that came her way. I remember her always looking strict and slightly forbidding when I was young, which may have had something to do with her spectacles and rather formal habit of dress, and she always seemed to be on the verge of disapproval. If she had need of anything, then she always acquired the biggest and best example of that object that she could. As mentioned, she owned the largest cooker that I had ever seen, more of a range really, which was probably fine in the kitchen of the guest house, but which took up a sizeable portion of the much smaller kitchen in the modern bungalow. Her refrigerator looked like those massive ones I saw on American television programmes rather than the smaller under-counter one our family had at home at the time. The refrigerator door had a long handle with a small lock built in beneath, and thick bulging sides, with cavernous interior, but there never seemed to be any spare space within for it was always crammed with food. Not that we would dare to ever help ourselves to anything within.

Steve and I also loved her car, which, true to form, was a Vauxhall Velox, a pale blue whale of a thing, with large leather bench seats front and back, a gear lever on the steering column and a speedometer that fascinated us. Rather than the usual circular dial around which a needle travelled to indicate the speed, this car had a horizontal meter with the speeds reading left to right, and a revolving cylinder painted in different colours which became apparent as the speed increased and the cylinder rotated. At lower speeds the colour displayed was green, slowly moving into amber as the speed rose up to the middle range. Needless to say, both Steve and I kept imploring our Nana to get up to the red end of the meter, which was really only possible on the nearby main road. This car also featured heavily in an incident long remembered in the family, when we had gone to the New Forest to see some of the semi-wild ponies there. The ponies, no doubt through experience, clearly recognised the car park as a place to get food and were not shy around humans or their motor vehicles. No sooner had Nana parked the car and opened her window for some fresh air, than a pony put its head right inside, presumably to see what was on offer, resulting in delighted shrieks from us children. What is more, once there, the pony showed no inclination to remove its head again. Having eventually been persuaded to do so it then began to gnaw at the outside door handle, covering it in drool, and then dropped a surprisingly large and aromatic pile of what Nana referred to as "rose fertiliser" in such a place that it was impossible to get out of the doors on the driver's side without running the risk of stepping into it. From then on, the sight of any accumulation of horse manure on the highway led to a comment to the effect that we should have brought a bucket to collect it in and take it back home to put on the roses.

Nana was also memorable for her collection of furs of which she was inordinately proud. She had coats and hats as well as a fox stole on which the head and paws of the poor creature were both present and obvious. Whilst these would mark her out in today's society and attract unwelcome attention and abuse, they were seen back then as desirable items usually owned by the well to do. The other noticeable thing was her standing within her community. She became chairwoman of the local Townswomen's Guild, and always seemed to be busy with meetings and committees. This only seemed to increase after Grandpa died and she had even more time to fill once relieved of her caring duties at home.

Family trips down to the South Coast to visit our grandparents became less frequent as we got into our teenage years, but there was one last occasion when the bungalow became a bolthole for me. I was revising for my A levels, probably too much and too intensely, often sitting up reading until I was unable to actually concentrate on the page any longer. All of this intensity brought on migraines, from which I had never previously suffered, but which Mum had and so she sympathised. Therefore, it was decided I needed a break from the studying and probably from the home environment as well. Dad always did the navigating, and this was at a time long before satellite navigation devices. He would therefore use an AA Book of the Road, which was not always up-to-date, and the various problems of him imparting the directions in time for Mum to respond to them have been alluded to earlier. However, he could not take the time off from work to be involved and so Mum and I went down by train and were met by Nana at the splendidly named Hinton Admiral station. We spent a very pleasant week near the South coast, with me doing some work, but mostly just getting away from the intensity of exam preparation and walking along the coast in the fresh air.

I can only remember three more visits to that part of the country after that. The first one was a large family gathering at Nana's ninetieth birthday, when Mum and her two sisters went with all their assorted children, all girls but for Steve and I as mentioned. The next was the funeral of Nana's brother, my godfather, who lived along the coast from Nana and whom I mostly remember for always being busy with his vegetable patch in the garden or pruning his roses. He had been unwell for a while by then, and he died leaving behind his wife of innumerable years. She was a feisty and determined lady despite being of diminutive stature. She had Indian heritage and a strong Welsh accent, and her dark and wrinkled skin made her look like a walnut to my eyes. She subsequently returned to her family in Wales to live out the rest of her own days. The last occasion for a visit was the funeral for

Nana herself a couple of years afterwards when, in her nineties, she finally succumbed to worsening heart failure that proved resistant to medical help. Despite those promises one makes to oneself over future intentions, I have not been to that part of the Country since. Mum keeps a photograph of her mother on the sideboard in her own dining room, where it is in the company of one or two pieces kept from Nana's own furniture and ornaments when she passed. The photo had been taken outside the front of the bungalow, with its distinctive stone façade framing the porch behind her, and whenever we visit, I always smile and say "Hi Nana" under my breath when I see it on the sideboard as I bend to retrieve the glasses for a pre-lunch sherry. So now that I am the Grandpa what I mostly want is to ensure that my grandsons' earliest memories of me, and those yet to come, are of comfort and security, like those I have of my own grandparents. I hope that the contact and input that I have can be little nuggets of gold that they can hold on to throughout their lives and polish up in their memories, so that they hopefully bring a rosy glow with them whenever they are recalled, together with fond memories and an affection that lasts the test of time. Whether there will be more grandchildren to come, from Mary or Rose or through any reconciliation with my other children, I do not know, but I do know that I would want to be a part of their life and a part that they would cherish. I have also at last come to understand myself and be comfortable with that. For so much of my life I have seemed not to fit in, and I could never understand why that was. My understanding of my own nature and the patterns of my behaviour that identify me are understandable and predictable now that the explanation for them is known. It has given me the freedom to accept that I just view things differently to others and that this world view is just as valid as anybody else's and does not need to be changed or revised to fit in with theirs. They have just as much need to make allowances for me as I have for them, and this realisation has also brought me an element of peace and understanding that had been missing for so much of my life. I now know what makes me tick, and I do not feel the need to analyse that further or try to change it. I need no validation from anybody else, though for many years that is exactly what I have sought. Rather than try to be a part of a group to identify with, I have realised that I have become content with the individual that I am. I like order and perspective, regularity and predictability. I like to count things for no particular reason, and it pleases me to do so somehow, whether it is slats in a fence or indentations on a radiator, and I find comfort and contentment in even numbers and symmetry. I like to play by the rules and have no time for those who do not. I do not feel the need to explain myself to those who don't understand me.

I will probably never really know why my children dropped me from their lives, but I have learned to compartmentalise that pain so that it has reduced with time. That elephant in the room whenever I am with Rose is still there, but it has shrunk to something much smaller that could fit neatly in a corner and be less intrusive. I do not feel fully at ease with her despite that, because without knowing why the estrangement happened, I cannot be fully confident that it will not happen again, and I want to protect myself from that potential pain. However, the joy of being with my grandsons outshines that small cloud, and I remain prepared to wait to see if Rose wants to address the issue. She has already stated that her biggest regret in life was not having me at her wedding and that it was something she could not ever put right. I can see no point in rubbing salt into that wound and other reflections may bring further comment from Rose on her behaviour in due course. As for my other two children, well I am a patient man and can wait. Rose has mentioned that Bradley has had some mental health problems since leaving university and I cannot help wondering whether he has been battling some of the same demons that I did at that age, given our similar personality traits. I only hope that he finds his own way to the same conclusions that I have, but hopefully much earlier in life.

I have never really sustained many friendships, only having one or two good friends at any one time. Whereas others might stay in touch with friends from school or university, or work colleagues, for many years, I never have. This seems to be by mutual, if unspoken, consent as nobody has tried to stay in touch with me either. When driving home from work on a Friday evening I generally listen to the drive time request show on the radio and hear about people traversing the country to meet up or travelling together as a group of friends who have known each other for years, but it is so far removed from my own experience that I cannot identify with what they are doing. There are also descriptions of parties for significant birthdays or anniversaries, and this is also outside of my experience or comfort zone. Apart from having such a small social circle that I could hold a party in a phone-box and still leave room for dancing, I hate being the centre of attention. I only managed to get through two weddings because the focus is on the bride and the main speech comes from the Best Man. All I really had to do was turn up sober, repeat the lines given to me, and smile a lot.

This is just a part of who I am. I have realised that it is not that I am "no fun," or a "stick-in-the-mud" or "a grumpy old sod," or, rather, I am only those things when seen through the eyes of people who do not share my idiosyncrasies. In reality, I am just trying my best to navigate what is, for me, a hostile environment. Because of my Asperger's, going to a party or function involving a room full of people I do not know is my worst nightmare as it overwhelms my ability to cope. This can be managed, if I can engage in small numbers, preferably involving somebody I already know, and limit the interactions. I am no good at small talk, and the worst thing I can be asked to do is to "circulate." However, I do want to be involved and to enjoy myself. After all, the next person one meets could be one who changes your life, you never know. I just have to go about it in a particular way. Perhaps that is why I like the company of my dogs so much. They all have different personalities and preferences themselves, but they ask nothing more than some attention, exercise, and food, in return for which they give unconditional love regardless of mood or circumstances. They, too, are creatures of habit and routine, with few expectations, a tendency towards predictability, and there is no side to them. They do not play the games that people play amongst themselves, and you always know exactly where you stand with them. I have realised that my tendency to wear my heart on my sleeve and to take things at face value has made me susceptible to the manipulative wiles of others and that I retreat as it is the only form of defence that I know. Being deceitful or economical with the truth makes me feel uneasy so I know I could not play such people at their own game, especially as there are so many people out there who play it much better.

How many of us ever take the time to truly reflect upon what makes us happy or unhappy or think about how we get on with others. By being secure in oneself there is no need to have those concerns and things become much more relaxed. I have always felt that I have been playing somebody else's game and by their rules for most of my life, and the understanding that this is not necessary has been the key to finding a different future and a hopefully more fulfilling way of life. If only I had made this discovery sooner things might have been different, but regret and ruminations are of no help. I have to accept the situation as it is and move forward, hoping that my new insight reduces the chance of me making the same mistakes again. There are no guarantees of a Happy Ever After, but contentment for the foreseeable future would suit me just fine. Some people have heard my explanations of how other people manipulate and condescend, and my concerns over the casual laziness of authority, and have called me cynical. All I can say in return is that what they consider to be cynicism is what I call life experience.

ACKNOWLEDGEMENT

This book has really been a solo effort, but I must thank my wife for her unstinting support and encouragement throughout the four years it took me to put this book together and get it into a form that I was happy to share. There will be more to come.

www.ingramcontent.com/pod-product-compliance
Lightning Source LLC
Chambersburg PA
CBHW052346220526
45465CB00003BA/977